GET SOBER, GET FREE

YOUR PRACTICAL GUIDE

VERONICA VALLI

Recovery Advocate and Recovered Alcoholic

Consultant Editor: Annemarie Young

Published by
Ebby Publishing
www.ebbypublishing.com

Disclaimer

The information contained in this book is based on the personal and
professional experiences of the author. It is not intended as a substi-
tute for consulting with your physician or other healthcare professional. The author and publisher are not responsible for any adverse side
effects or consequences resulting directly or indirectly from the use
of any of the suggestions discussed in this book. All matters pertain-
ing to your individual health should be supervised by a healthcare professional. Some of the names and locations of the people and clients
mentioned in this book have been changed to protect their identity.

About the Author

Veronica Valli, Recovery Advocate, NLP Prac, Ad Dip, MASC Life Coach, EFT Prac

Veronica is the author of the best-selling book *Why You Drink and How to Stop*. She runs a popular blog http://veronicavalli.com where she regularly writes about issues relating to alcoholism and addiction.

As a recovered alcoholic and drug addict, she has personal experience of what it takes to recover from an addiction. Veronica struggled with alcoholism through most of her twenties. As a binge drinker, she was aware for some time that something was wrong but was unable to define what it was; a chance meeting led to her finally getting help and turning her life around.

At the height of her addiction, Veronica was unable to go to work without the aid of a drink; her life and confidence were in tatters. She got sober in 2000 at the age of twenty-seven. She now uses this experience to help and inspire others. She fully believes that all alcoholics and addicts can recover if they have access to the right kind of help, and that they can then go on to live life to the full.

She is committed to educating and informing the public on problem drinking and addiction and has appeared regularly on BBC Radio Cambridgeshire as a specialist guest. She has appeared on the Lorraine

Kelly show on ITV, and an ITV programme entitled *The Truth About Binge Drinking*; she has also appeared in national magazines and publications, discussing recovery from alcoholism.

Veronica is married with two young sons.

http://veronicavalli.com
http://twitter.com/veronicavalli
https://www.facebook.com/addictionexpert

About the Consultant Editor

Annemarie Young, Writer and publishing consultant, BAHons, DipEd, MSc, MA

Annemarie has worked in publishing for almost thirty years: as a senior editor in a major university publishing house in the UK for the first twenty years, and after that as an editorial consultant for a number of large publishers.

She also writes books for young children learning to read, is co-author of an acclaimed non-fiction series for older children, and co-author with Michael Rosen of a book on Humanism for older children. She is a Senior Member at a University of Cambridge graduate college.

Praise for *Why You Drink and How to Stop*

Kristen Johnston, two-time Emmy award winning actress, NYT Best Selling Author and Recovery Advocate, says:

> *"Veronica Valli has written one of the clearest, most fascinating and truly helpful books on addiction I've ever read.*
>
> *To me, it's up there with* Clean *by David Sheff, except from the viewpoint of someone who's in long-term recovery.*
>
> *Whether you're struggling now and need help, have struggled in the past, or you've ever loved an addict, this book pierces through the confusing and terrifying misinformation that surrounds this disease.*
>
> *From the first page to the last, I was completely enthralled by this brilliantly researched, refreshingly straightforward and delightfully compelling book."*

Dedication

This book is dedicated to:
every addict and alcoholic I have ever known
and to Lukey who is joy beyond anything I could have
imagined.

Acknowledgements

As usual I would like to thank my editor Annemarie Young – your professionalism and dedication to perfection inspire me all the time. I am so lucky to be able to work with such a talented and wonderful woman. I will always be in your debt.

And thank you to Hilary Ratcliff, our copy editor, for your meticulous attention to detail.

I also owe thanks to my darling husband who leans in whenever he can, is an amazing father to our gorgeous boys and is my biggest cheerleader and fan. Thank you for always believing in me.

I would lastly like to thank everyone who has written to me or contacted me regarding my first book and blog. Your comments and praise have inspired me beyond anything you will ever know. You do not struggle alone; we struggle along this wonderful road of sobriety together. You are the stars that light the way.

Contents

CONTENTS

Introduction

I N MY BOOK *Why You Drink and How to Stop* I explore why feelings and emotions are the engine that drive destructive drinking. The key to overcoming an alcohol problem lies in understanding how to manage and interpret our feelings, deal with our past and develop strategies to manage our present circumstances no matter what they are.

Through my blog http://veronicavalli.com and social media I have interacted with many people who have read my book and benefited from its advice. Many people have asked me what work they can specifically do in order to successfully recover from their drinking problem. This is exactly what this workbook is about. It takes you through a variety of exercises that invite you to look deeper into the reasons behind your drinking and goes on to help you develop successful recovery strategies that ensure your sobriety has a firm foundation.

These are strategies and methods that I have used personally and with clients in over a decade of experience working with addicts and alcoholics.

I'll be honest with you – some of these questions will be difficult to answer, but it's vitally important that you do. As I explain in *Why You Drink and How to Stop*, if stopping drinking was as simple as putting down the drink and not picking one up again, no one would have a problem. Unfortunately, the reasons behind our destructive drinking patterns are much more pervasive and complicated than that. The primary reason we drink is because it works at one level. Alcohol is a very powerful anaesthetic that prevents us from feeling unpleasant or uncomfortable feelings; it completely blocks out things we don't want to face and comforts the fear and uneasiness that threatens to overwhelm us. It also takes away our dignity, integrity, motivation; it robs us of our ambition and ability to achieve our full potential. When we let alcohol dominate us, we live a 50% life and become shadows of the people we could have been.

Is this you?

If it is you then I need to ask: are you done yet?

Because if you are, then I wrote this book for you. I'm aware that not everyone can afford, or is able to go to, a 28-day treatment programme, or is able see a therapist of some kind. If those options are at all possible for you, I would strongly urge you to pursue them. If you are preparing to go into treatment or seek help with a professional, you will find this book extremely helpful in your treatment.

If you are not able to seek any professional help at this point, then this book will support you in the next steps of your sobriety journey. The most important thing I want you to know is that you are not alone. Many others have walked this path of loneliness and despair, and there is a way out.

How this book works

This book is divided into different sections. The first section deals with looking at your drinking patterns and how you use alcohol. The second section looks at the feelings and emotions that are driving your drinking, and what areas of your life you need to clean up in order to stay sober. The last section looks at our sober goals and strategies to ensure we are living the best life possible.

Each section of the book has questions you need to answer. Writing your answers will be extremely powerful. I strongly urge that you write down your answers instead of just answering them in your head. It is enormously therapeutic to begin to extract the stuff that has been whirling around inside us and put it on paper. It makes things real. It's actually harder to lie to ourselves or deny what is going on when we see it on paper in front of us. Successfully overcoming alcoholism requires us to be honest. This may be frightening at first but in the long term it is a much easier way to live.

If you have someone you trust and can share your answers with them, you may find it useful to read out loud what you have written.

Sharing what is really going on with us, rather than the obligatory 'I'm fine', is also enormously healing. If you don't have someone you can talk with, then you will still get enormous benefit from writing the answers out.

Don't try to do the exercises in a couple of days. Recovery is going to take a little longer than that. I'd suggest doing one section a week. Take your time; the more you write the better. The point of the work is to really absorb your answers whilst working on staying sober.

A WORD OF CAUTION

If you are alcohol *dependent,* meaning you are physically dependent on alcohol, then it is extremely unsafe for you to stop drinking without a medical intervention of some kind. Alcohol is far more dangerous to detox from than say, heroin, because the sufferer could die if not properly supported (this isn't necessarily the case with a heroin detox; it's extremely unpleasant, but not usually dangerous if managed). It is very, very important if you are a regular, heavy drinker that you seek medical help if you want to stop.

You can do this in many ways. The first step would be to go and see your doctor. You can then be referred to a local specialist service, or be prescribed medication that will enable you to detox from alcohol safely. Your doctor should be the best resource for what support and treatment are available to you locally. If you are in bad physical shape then it may be appropriate that you enter an in-patient facility where you will receive full medical care. This is to prevent withdrawal symptoms like seizures, restlessness and arrhythmia from becoming life threatening. It can also help relieve the symptoms of anxiety, restlessness and insomnia that often accompany the first few days of alcohol withdrawal. *It is essential you seek professional medical help that can assess what is the best option for you.*

Supporting your sobriety

If you have made the decision to quit drinking and have heeded the advice about how to stop if you are physically dependent, then you are ready to start work on the reasons behind your drinking. Whilst going through this workbook there are other things you can be doing that support your sobriety:

- Consider joining a self-help group to meet other sober people.
- Join an on-line support group for people with alcohol problems.
- Tell your health care provider what you are doing.
- Exercise regularly.
- Try eating healthier foods.
- Get as much sleep as you can.
- Avoid friends who drink and 'wet' places for the time being.
- Tell a supportive friend what you are doing.

Section 1

Honesty

What are my drinking patterns?

WE ARE GOING to start by looking at your relationship with alcohol. As problem drinkers we often fudge the details and consequences of our drinking. Alcoholics and problem drinkers are masters of rationalising their drinking and pretending it's 'normal'. The purpose of this exercise is to get the facts on paper, so there's no escaping them. The decision to stop drinking must be followed by action. By completing these exercises you are taking action towards sustaining your sobriety. Because alcohol abuse has been so normalised in our culture, it's very difficult for us to accept that we ourselves have a problem. We tend to measure ourselves against extreme examples and because we don't meet those extremes we convince ourselves that our drinking is 'normal' or at least not harmful. We need to let go of all of those preconceived ideas and really look closely at how alcohol affects us.

In many ways it's quite simple. Every problem drinker asks themselves the same question at a certain point: am I an alcoholic or not?

That's the million-dollar question, isn't it?

It's the question many people who drink to excess find themselves asking at some point or another.

Could I be an alcoholic? A sinking feeling in your stomach, followed by a desperate scramble to try to reassure yourself that you're not, usually follows this thought. I know, because I've done it. When I was going to college and drinking vodka in the toilets before a 9am lecture it occurred to me that this is what alcoholics do. My stomach lurched in fear and I thought to myself, 'No, I can't be an alcoholic, because alcoholics enjoy drinking alcohol and I'm only drinking because I have to.'

I used to get really bad panic attacks and the only thing that really worked in calming them was booze. At twenty-three years old I couldn't be in a group situation sober so I really struggled in college and work environments where I couldn't drink. I would often nip to the pub at lunchtime and have a drink or two to get me through the afternoon. Not enough to get drunk; just enough to calm the fear and enable me to function.

But I was no good if I had to do any kind of group activity in the morning. I had to go to college and I had to go to work. These things were important so I had to find a way to get through without having a panic attack. Prescription drugs only ever seemed to work for a while. Booze was the only thing I could rely on.

Which is why, in my desperation to rationalise that I wasn't an alcoholic, I came up with the conclusion that I wasn't an alcoholic, as I was drinking out of *necessity*.

Of course now I can see how crazy that is. But the truth is that I actually had no idea what an alcoholic really was. I thought it was a smelly old man on a bench. I thought there were certain criteria that you needed to fulfill in order to be classed an alcoholic. I was certain that homelessness was one of them, and I was a college student for goodness sake. So I was definitely not an alcoholic.

I was wrong.

I was in full-blown alcoholism and it took me four more years to see this. I resisted right till the end because I was never physically addicted to alcohol, and I thought physical addiction was definitely one of the criteria for defining an alcoholic. I couldn't see that I was psychologically addicted and that my whole life was defined by drink. When that last delusion was stripped from me, I had nowhere left to hide.

Still unable to accept the truth, someone told me something that changed my life. They said alcoholics do three things:

- They drink.
- They think about drinking.
- They think about not drinking.

Oh wow, that was me. Right there. That was all the definition I needed. I was an alcoholic. And strangely, the feeling that followed that admission was actually relief. Because when I finally accepted and realised what my problem actually was, it meant I could finally start doing something about it. It was when I started doing something about my problem that everything changed.

If you are still having that debate with yourself then the following questions are designed to help you decide if you have a drinking problem.

Activity – How bad is my drinking problem?

1. At what age did you first try alcohol?
2. Can you remember the first time you got drunk? Describe what happened.
3. Do you ever drink on your own? How often?
4. Do you have a group of friends with whom you drink? How often?
5. How often do you drink alcohol?
6. How often are you hung over?
7. How do hangovers affect your life?

Think of the last few times you used alcohol or drugs. How did you feel in the hours before picking up?

1. What body sensations did you feel?
2. Did you have any physical discomfort, pain or agitation?
3. Could you concentrate?
4. Describe how you usually respond to these sensations.

About cravings

Cravings can take place before or after we start to use a substance. Our thinking tends to get pre-occupied by the thought of drinking; this is the stage before drinking when we usually feel excited and look forward to how alcohol is going to make us feel. If we are feeling negative, we are looking forward to the numbness that alcohol can bring. There are *two* types of cravings:

1. One kind of craving takes place *before* the first drink or hit. In this case, our feelings become signals to start drinking. The events or places that signal these feelings are called *triggers.*
2. The other kind of craving comes *after* the first drink. Once we start drinking, we crave more. For example, most people stop after having one or two drinks. But after one or two drinks, active alcoholics are just getting started. Despite their intentions, alcoholics tend to lose control over how much they drink once they start.

Knowing the difference between these two kinds of cravings can help you deal with these urges.

Activity – Triggers

Think about your personal triggers, or your signals to pick up a drink. List some of your triggers.

1. Are there certain people, places or things that make you think about drinking? For instance walking into a pub is an obvious one.
2. Are there certain days that make you feel like drinking?
3. Or certain events, like particular sports?
4. What about people? Who are the people you always end up drinking with?

Taking action to prevent cravings

There are different kinds of myths about cravings. One myth is that cravings come out of nowhere and there's little you can do about them. Another myth is that you'll die or go crazy unless you give in to a craving. Some people even think that just feeling a craving or giving in to one means that their recovery is dead. Actually, none of these myths is true. As you deal with cravings, keep in mind that:

- Cravings are usually triggered by certain sights, sounds, smells, people, places or things. We can prevent cravings by avoiding unnecessary triggers – this is especially necessary when we are first trying to get sober. I'm over fifteen years sober now and I can safely go into a pub to eat and socialise without ever thinking about alcohol, but it was not something I could do straight away. We can also learn to have different responses to our triggers. This is where outside support is particularly helpful as it's often hard to deal with these powerful cravings on our own.

▪ Cravings can lead to a lot of discomfort, but they are not fatal. When we consistently abstain, our cravings will gradually fade over time. And they will eventually disappear altogether.

▪ Generally it's *actions* that will change things rather than trying to *think* your way out of a craving. The key here is to *do* something. Take a walk, call a friend, ask for help.

Activity – Cravings

1. Look again at your list of triggers and list ways you can prevent them turning into cravings.
2. Brainstorm ways to change your reaction to the people, places and things that trigger cravings (eg does an argument with your wife always lead to your walking out and going to the pub)?
3. What can you do differently?

Drinking to deal with feelings

Many of us have a history of stress, pain or abuse. In some cases our background includes physical abuse, sexual abuse, rape or incest. Often we came from families where one or more members were substance dependent. Maybe we just weren't parented well and our emotional needs were not adequately met, and we felt lonely, isolated or just different from other people. Often we were *scared* of other people.

Some of us responded to the pain and stress in our lives by using substances. But pain and stress do not *cause* us to become dependent or abuse alcohol or drugs. The drugs or alcohol may have eased or distracted us from pain, fear or anger, but many people go through painful experiences *without* using alcohol or other drugs. We, on the other hand, started abusing alcohol or drugs and found we couldn't stop using them.

Using alcohol or drugs to deaden emotional pain and deal with fear is something *we learn how to do.*

There are more appropriate ways of dealing with our negative emotions and fears, and recovery is about learning some of those ways.

Activity – Feelings

1. Describe two situations when you have been in emotional pain or felt fear and have responded by using alcohol or drugs. What were you thinking and how did you feel *before*, *during* and *after* you picked up? Be specific.
2. Is there a particular feeling you can't cope with that always leads you to drink?
3. Is there a particular situation that you find difficult that you always use alcohol to cope with?

The answers to these questions will reveal how you *rely* on alcohol to cope. Which means it has gone from something you find pleasurable to being a crutch. If alcohol is our crutch then it is not something that is going to help. There are better ways to deal with feelings and situations we find challenging.

What has drinking cost me?

Activity – Financial cost

How much (in money) has your alcohol use cost you in your lifetime? Get a piece of paper and a calculator and do a rough 'guesstimate' of the financial toll of your alcohol use.
(Consider: lost jobs or work, fines, moving, lost opportunities, medical bills, broken or lost possessions, divorces, childcare, debts, actual cost of alcohol.)

This figure can be quite sobering (literally!). At first we may think we just waste money on buying alcohol but this is rarely the case. Consider how many times you end up ordering a take-away instead of cooking, or ordering a taxi instead of driving. Have you ever lost or ruined an item of clothing whilst out drinking? What about lost productivity? Has your earning potential diminished due to your alcohol problem? How much have you lost in potential earnings? Has a marriage ended because of your drinking problem? How much did the divorce cost you?

When we examine it closely, we are sometimes shocked to see the actual financial cost of our drinking. This isn't the only cost but sometimes seeing a figure in pounds or dollars makes us sit up and take notice.

The harder part is looking at what our drinking problem has cost us in other ways.

Activity – Cost to relationships

How has alcohol affected the relationships with people you love? Describe how alcohol has damaged your relationships.

1. Have you compromised your integrity or morals due to alcohol? (Have you lied, manipulated or deceived people because of your drinking? Have you done something while drunk that you would never consider doing while sober, and that you look back on in horror?)
2. What is at risk if you don't stop drinking?
3. Have you tried to quit drinking before? What happened?
4. How have you lied to yourself about your drinking?

What scares you about not drinking again? Let's face it, alcohol has been our best friend; it's always been there for us. We've relied on it totally to deal with any situation or emotion that scares us. It's not that we don't want to get sober and change our lives; it's just that the thought of living without the crutch of alcohol terrifies us.

I want you to know that's perfectly natural. Every single person who has quit alcohol because of a drinking problem has felt the same way. There is a way to fill the hole that alcohol used to fill, and there are methods and strategies that can be applied that will enable us to live the life the way we were meant to. But to get there we have to take each day as it comes. As each week goes by you will find life gets easier and easier.

If you are putting the effort into this and answering these questions honestly, then I'm guessing you probably feel pretty bad about yourself right now.

Stop that immediately. I want to assure you that you are not a bad person, just a sick one. It's also very important for you to understand that you are not alone. Every single person with an alcohol problem feels the same way. We have all done things we are completely ashamed about. We can all look back at our behaviour in horror because it's so far away from the people we really are.

We are not writing this stuff down to feel bad about ourselves; we are writing it down so that we can heal, leave it in the past and move on unburdened.

In many ways alcoholism is self-perpetuating: we drink to make ourselves feel better, then we do something we regret or feel awful about, so we then drink more to forget about it. And so it goes on.

If you read my blog, veronicavalli.com, you will see that every week I interview someone in recovery who has overcome their drinking and turned their lives around. I have interviews with mothers who have almost killed their children whilst driving drunk, people who have been homeless and abandoned by their families, and people who have suffered enormous abuse. All of these people have managed to overcome their drinking and found new ways to live. Please check out their stories as you will then see you are no worse than anyone else, and know that if they can change their lives then you can too!

There is only one thing I want you to focus on right now and that is how incredibly brave you are. What you are doing is immensely courageous. This is the real you. Please focus on that aspect of yourself. As difficult as it is to answer these questions, you may find that just by getting this stuff on paper you actually feel slightly better. The reason for this is that all of these thoughts and feelings have been fermenting inside you. Getting them out is the first part in moving on from them.

Internal and external unmanageability

Now I want to look at the internal and external unmanageability that alcohol abuse can cause. (This comes from *Why You Drink and How to Stop*.)

The unmanageability of alcoholism can present itself in numerous ways:
- Unpaid bills
- Debt
- Broken relationships
- Broken promises
- Drink driving
- Criminal charges
- Fraud
- Neglect of children
- Neglect of self
- Unexplained accidents
- Loss of personal possessions
- Problems at work
- Getting fired from jobs
- Leaving jobs before getting fired
- Disorganisation
- Losing things
- Physical injury
- Bad timekeeping
- Memory loss
- Homelessness
- Violence.

The list is really endless. The bottom line is that when someone is drinking alcohol to excess, their life becomes chaotic. They can't stay on top of things. They can't keep commitments. They are consistently unreliable. As their drinking progresses, the consequences usually become more serious.

But there is also another level of unmanageability, and that is *emotional unmanageability*. To some degree, the alcoholic may be able to create some sense of order in their outside world. They may be able to work and pay their mortgage, for instance. This is how some alcoholics can convince themselves they don't have a problem; because they have a job and a car they believe that things can't be that bad. However, their emotional life is completely unmanageable, and by that I mean *they have no control over how they are going to feel*. Using alcohol gives them the false illusion that they have control over their feelings, when the opposite is actually true.

They succumb to depression and irritability; they have a constant feeling of dissatisfaction. They get angry over small issues; they constantly resent other people for what they do or say. They are unhappy. Small things upset them and they over-react.

Emotional unmanageability is when you have no control over how you are going to feel or react at any particular time.

If you have no control over how you feel, then your feelings lead you, and you become a slave to them. Being in charge of your emotional life, rather than the other way round, is essential to long term recovery.

How is my life unmanageable?

Let's identify how your life is unmanageable due to alcohol.

Activity – Unmanageable life

1. Give three examples where your alcohol use has caused something negative to happen in your life. (eg Did you get fired because you were constantly late for work due to hangovers? Have you repeatedly lost your wallet and had to cancel credit cards on a regular basis? Have you missed an opportunity because you just didn't have your act together?)
2. Have you let a loved one or friend down because you were drunk or hung-over? If so, what happened?

For some of us, we managed to run our lives fairly well whilst still drinking destructively. We kept our jobs, we never got caught drinking and driving, we turned up (mostly) when we had to, but inside we were just falling apart.

Now let's look at how our emotions and feelings have been unmanageable and how we've used alcohol to manage them.

Activity – Unmanageable emotions

Think about a recent time when you felt angry/frightened/disturbed in some way.

What happened? Was it an incident at work or at home? Did nothing happen but you've just woken up feeling down or upset and thought a drink might help you feel better?

Describe in detail a time when you used alcohol to numb unpleasant feelings. What were the consequences? How did you feel after?

We often use alcohol to control our feelings because we haven't developed a more healthy or productive way of dealing with feelings that every human being has to deal with. In sobriety we need to learn more effective ways of dealing with disappointment, fear, rejection and so on. We will be looking at how to do that in Section 3.

What help is available to me?

There are many methods and routes to getting sober. Some people find going to meetings of Alcoholics Anonymous is tremendously helpful; others have found Cognitive Behavioural Therapy (CBT) very useful. There are numerous types of therapy, rehabs and support groups that can offer help to someone trying to recover from alcoholism.

Your chances of success can be greatly increased if you plug into some kind of support. Research what is available to you locally. Are there any free support services? What paid services are there?

Ensure that you work with reputable therapists: check they are accredited and/or licensed and insured. Personal recommendations are always good.

Be open-minded and try different approaches. The chances are that you will find a group, therapist or approach that you feel comfortable and safe with. But you may have to spend some time exploring what your options are.

Problem drinkers have a tendency to isolate and withdraw, so it's important that you push yourself out of your comfort zone and endeavour to stay connected to people who can help you.

What is my abstinence date?

Activity – Abstinence date

Record in your diary your first day of being alcohol free.

This is the first day of the rest of your life, so remember and cherish it.

Summary

Deciding to stop drinking is a big step; it can be scary and confusing. In order to establish successful, sustainable sobriety we must be prepared to really examine our drinking patterns. Because abnormal drinking has become so normalised in our culture, we often minimise how bad our drinking is because we can always think of someone who is worse than we are. We can rationalise away the consequences of our drinking and continue to live in denial.

But if we have answered the previous questions honestly then we will have begun to see a pattern emerge. By pulling all the pieces of the puzzle together, we can see the whole picture for the first time. We have revealed to ourselves how much alcohol has cost us financially, and also emotionally. We will also have discovered that we just haven't fulfilled our potential, and even though we *thought* our drinking was under control, we have discovered that it impacted our lives and other people's far more deeply than we may have believed.

The level of honesty you have just achieved is remarkable. Even though these exercises may have been difficult and uncomfortable, they are the pathways to freedom. It's our shame and secrets that burden us. Today you are breaking chains. Take a moment to congratulate yourself on your honesty and the enormous step you have taken. You have done something you should be proud of.

Section 2

Reality

I N THIS SECTION we are going to explore the underlying reasons for your drinking.

As I wrote in *Why You Drink and How to Stop*:

We behave how we feel

Everyone, whether or not they are alcoholics, has positive and negative feelings and then acts upon those feelings. All behaviour is dictated by how we feel; we act emotionally. We may think we make rational decisions but how we feel always takes precedence. Just look around and you will see that this is true. Now here is the catch: if your emotions are unmanageable, and you have no control over when or why you feel negative emotions, then these emotions will dictate how you behave. This is because when we feel bad we are motivated to get rid of that feeling as quickly and as effectively as possible. And alcohol is a powerful anaesthetic for negative emotions.

The behaviour of an alcoholic makes sense to them at the time

So, with some understanding of how alcoholics really feel and what is actually motivating them, it becomes easier to understand why alcoholics behave the way they do.

From the outside an alcoholic's behaviour can seem to be that of a lunatic. I can assure you, *to them*, at the time, their behaviour makes perfect sense – because it is based on how they feel. One of the worst things about a descent into alcoholism is the realisation that you are behaving in a way that isn't *you*.

Our drinking behaviour is just a manifestation of feelings that we cannot express, or process, in healthier and more productive ways. In order to achieve successful, sustainable sobriety we *have to* deal with the root causes and that means we have to understand how and why we feel the way we do.

For me, this was a very scary thought. I had, after all, spent a lifetime running away from how I felt. I used alcohol to put a lid on any feelings. I wanted to be numb. I was very, very frightened at the thought of having to finally explore what I'd been running away from.

So if you are feeling the same way, I want you to know that is perfectly normal. The following questions and strategies are designed to help you explore those feelings in a way that is comfortable. You may find that when you begin the process of revealing yourself to yourself, the reality of understanding and experiencing your emotions is far less scary than the thought of actually doing it. Sometimes reality is easier.

Liabilities and assets

If it were as easy as just stopping drinking, we would all just stop drinking as soon as we realised we had a problem.

But it isn't that easy, is it?

Which is why we need to look at how we are working *against* ourselves. Because in many ways we are our own worst enemy. If we have made the decision to get sober then we have to look at our liabilities, the parts of our character that hold us back. When someone has an alcohol problem, they usually have pretty low self-esteem, for instance. Low self-esteem will have an enormous impact on our choices and actions.

We don't want to over-focus on the negative stuff, so we are also going to look at your assets – the parts of your personality that work for you – and see how we can build on those strengths.

But let's get the ugly stuff out of the way first and look at liabilities. Remember this is not about beating ourselves up; it's about taking a good honest look at ourselves so we can move forward into a better future.

In 'recovery speak' this is sometimes known as 'character defects'. But I'm not keen on the term 'defects' as it's so negative. It really is just looking at parts of our character that work *against* us rather than *for* us.

Pride

The first liability is pride. We all suffer from too much pride and it always trips us up. This process is not about getting rid of all of these parts of ourselves; it's about getting them *in balance*. It's totally fine to feel pride for what we have achieved; what harms us is when we let pride *govern* us. Let me explain what pride really is: pride is the fear of what we *think* other people think about us. Ponder that one for a moment.

You have absolutely no *idea* what other people think about you. None. Yet we will make decisions and take actions based on how we *think* other people may react, or how we *think* they will feel towards us.

Everybody wants to be liked, that is a natural human need. However, it's a fact that not everyone will like us. *We are just not everyone's cup of tea.*

I know I'm not.

Not everyone who meets me, likes me. However, enough people do and that's really all that matters. I have not always felt this way. Back when I was drinking I would turn cartwheels to try to get people to like me. Often it was people I didn't like very much myself, but for some totally crazy reason, it really mattered to me that they thought I was 'something'. Because according to my crazy logic, if enough people thought I was 'something' then surely it would mean I actually was.

My pride also meant I could never ask for help and I could never ever admit I was vulnerable. Those things terrified me. I wanted you to believe the best of me, and if I admitted I was really struggling then surely you would see the worst of me, and that was something I could not bear.

So I created a prison for myself based on pride. Have you done the same?

Believe me that is not a successful way to live. Being able to live free of the good or bad opinion of other people is true freedom. Because then I started to like myself. I realised that when I tried to be the person I *thought* other people wanted, I was miserable and hated who I had become (hence the drinking). When I sobered up and started living my truth, I realised that the most important thing was that I should like myself.

Activity – Overcoming pride

Answer the following questions and let's look at how pride has chained you.

1. What decisions have you made based on what you thought other people would think? Have you made a decision because you wanted to please other people, or because you thought they would like you better because of your decision? How did it work out? Give details and examples.
2. Has your pride (fear of what other people think) ever prevented you from asking for help? How? What happened?
3. What frightens you about making a choice or taking an action that other people might not approve of?

Now let's look at the other side of pride. Let's look at accomplishments that you can be proud of. For example, I am extremely proud of my first book *Why You Drink and How to Stop*. Proud that I wrote it, got it published and it hit the number one slot in the alcoholism category for Amazon. I'm unbelievably proud of that. That's just one example of some things in my life that I am proud of. We can allow ourselves to feel proud of something we've worked hard to achieve!

Activity – Achievements to be proud of

What achievements are you proud of? Large or small, it doesn't matter.

Self-pity

Now let's look at the toxic emotion of self-pity. Self-pity is when we get 'stuck' in the story of 'It's not fair; look at all the awful things that have happened to me'. It's true many of us have had terrible things happen to us, and it wasn't fair and in many cases it wasn't our fault either. I don't want to minimise any of the terrible events you may have experienced, as they are valid experiences and your pain matters. What I want to do is help you to move past them so that you can be free of them. Self-pity is very 'heavy', it really weighs us down and makes us unattractive to people. Our story of woe dominates us and we lose who we really are.

Please understand that I am not saying you need to forget some terrible event or abuse that happened to you and become instantly perky and positive at all times. If something awful has happened, then get some support to move past it. Process what you can learn from what happened so you can be free of it. This may take time and you will probably need some outside help. But I want you to know you are not your story, you are so much more than that. And sometimes our story just holds us down.

Activity – Self-pity

1. Do you have a 'story' that you repeat to people that explains or excuses your drinking?
2. Who would you be without this 'story'?
3. What do you need to do to be free of the power of this 'story'?

Our 'story' is *part of* who we are, but it is not *who* we are. Who you are is not *what* happened to you, but how you choose to respond to what happened to you. In many ways our drinking was how we responded to what happened to us, and we didn't even realise that we were using alcohol to deal with our pain. Sobriety is how we choose a different response.

Selfishness

Booze and drugs make us unbelievably selfish – that's just a fact. We become incredibly self-centered, only thinking of our own wants and needs and completely ignoring or marginalising other people's feelings.

This next bit of self-analysis is going to be uncomfortable, but it's necessary that we recognise where we have been selfish so that we can begin to consider others more. Often, it hasn't really occurred to us that our behaviour has been selfish and that we have hurt other people by acting the way we have.

Activity – Selfishness

1. Describe how you have been selfish in your behaviour and actions due to your drinking.
2. What have been the consequences?
3. Can you remember a time when you didn't consider someone else's feelings or needs? What could you do differently?

Dishonesty

Dishonesty comes in many different packages. We can lie outright, which many of us do to cover up the reality of our drinking. Or we can withhold information, which is just another form of lying. Or we can have 'hidden agendas' where we say and do one thing in order to manipulate people into doing what we want.

We hide parts of ourselves and don't reveal our true motives or feelings; we say one thing and mean the other. These are all forms of dishonesty. Being dishonest often becomes a habit and this way of living often becomes second nature. Dishonesty with ourselves and other people is anxiety provoking – we always have to remember lies and stories we have told. We constantly feel like we are going to get found out. This is an uncomfortable way to live, and as I explored in my previous book, if we are in emotional pain for too long, then eventually we will seek something to numb it, and for us, that is usually alcohol.

So the path to sobriety means we have to begin to practise honesty with others and ourselves. It's a scary thought, isn't it? I know I felt terrified at the thought of not lying any more, or creating the kind of 'smoke and mirrors' dishonesty I was used to. Being honest can be hard, but it is certainly no harder than living a dishonest life, and the more you practise, the easier it gets.

Activity – Dishonesty

Try answering the following questions and pay attention to how you feel when you do.

1. How have you been dishonest recently? Have you kept certain information to yourself or misled someone? What happened? How did you feel?
2. Who can you begin to be honest with about your drinking?
3. In what ways have you been lying to yourself?
4. How have you manipulated other people? How did you feel when you were doing this?

Impatience

Impatience is when we want everything the way we want it NOW! It's a form of self-will, where we become bulldozers instead of people, and just push our agenda through regardless of other people's wants or concerns. When we are impatient, we take everything personally and perceive every delay as a slight on ourselves. We have an exaggerated sense of our own self-importance because we believe that our goals and needs take precedence over everyone else's. The way we see it is that it doesn't matter if we are rude, late or ignore people, because we need to do what we need to do and other people should understand that.

We are often impatient and angry when we want to drink or get drugs. This makes us extremely unpleasant to be around.

Activity – Impatience

1. When do you notice yourself getting impatient?
2. How does your impatience manifest itself? Do you shout, get angry?
3. How does this behaviour affect other people?

When we are caught up in our agenda, we often miss out on life and what is happening in the moment. We also miss our connection with other people, which just heightens our feelings of aloneness.

Jealousy/Envy

There is nothing so poisonous to the soul as feeling jealous. There is nothing more awful than that feeling that someone else has got something you should have had. In many ways, jealousy is just an extension of fear. The fear that we are going to 'miss out' or not get what we want. It also feeds our low self-esteem with feelings of 'it's not fair' and 'why can't I get what I want?'

Like our other liabilities, these feelings will begin to dissipate once we stop drinking and start becoming honest with ourselves.

Activity – Jealousy

1. When do you notice yourself feeling jealous or envious?
2. How do you behave when you feel jealous?

What are my fears?

In *Why You Drink and How to Stop* I wrote:

Nobody feels fear the way alcoholics feel fear
I'm aware that's not exactly true. However, there's something about alcoholic thinking that twists all our emotions and makes

the unpleasant ones dominant in us. We seem to take fear to a whole new level, much more than ordinary people do. It's like I was born frightened and my whole life has been a reaction to the fear. None of my fears were real, they were always imagined, but they seemed real to me and they followed me wherever I went. It was like a cancer of the mind, spreading and destroying everything in its path.

Fear is a massive liability and will dominate our lives and thinking more than anything else. I believe that fear is the engine that drives alcoholism and if we continue to let it dominate us then we will drink again. Alcohol numbs the fear allowing us to cope; if we want to get sober and stay sober then we have to find a better way of managing our fear. I believe one of the most effective ways of doing that is by beginning to be honest about our fears in the first place. Often we are just running away from them and the reality of facing them is far easier than running.

Activity – Fear

Answer the following questions as honestly as possible.

1. Make a list of all your fears. Include things like spiders and snakes, but the ones we are really looking for are things like 'fear of not being good enough', 'fear of other people', 'fear of not being loved'. These are more existential fears; they haunt us and have been around for as long as we can remember.
2. What frightens you about not drinking again? This is a very real fear for many people. Even though we may have accepted that alcohol is the cause of all our problems, it's still very hard for us to think of life without our crutch.
3. Who would you be, what would you do, if these fears didn't dominate your life?

Fear is the feeling we get when we believe that what is or is not going to happen will be disastrous for us, or harm us. This fear manifests itself as phobia, terror, panic, anxiety, worry or stress. When we are living and acting in fear we are trying to control the world so that we don't feel scared. This allows the fear to grow and take over our lives.

By listing our fears we have made a huge step towards challenging the power they have over us. In Section 3 we are going to look more closely at how we can have mastery over our emotions.

Activity – Liabilities

1. Look at all of your liabilities closely and identify which one has caused you the most problems in your life.
2. Can you give examples of where your pride or fear has caused negative outcomes?

The purpose of answering these questions is so we can convince ourselves that it's time to do something about our liabilities.

Everyone has defects and assets and it is important to recognise this. We need to be aware of our defects and how we 'indulge' in them, and we must also be aware of our assets, as acting on these will raise our self-esteem and enable our sense of worthiness to grow and flourish.

Our personalities are made up of the mental habits that we have accumulated, practised and now made into a fixed pattern. The problem is that we have developed many patterns that do not serve us; in fact they ultimately harm us.

By minimising our liabilities and focusing on our assets, we will develop behaviours that will serve us. We can always override anything in our life that is objectionable to us by using other, better ideas. When one of our old ways of thinking comes up (eg selfishness, greed), we will now be far more aware that this is something objectionable and harmful and therefore something that must go.

Assets

Now it's time to look at our assets. It's very easy for us to stay in a negative place and wallow in our own negativity. The purpose of identifying our liabilities is so we can be free of them and replace them with our assets. This doesn't mean we will ever become perfect but we can, in time, get more balanced and balance is the key to happiness.

Activity – Assets

The following is a list of character assets. Pick five which apply to you, and number them in order of significance.

- Grateful
- Tolerant
- Accepting
- Honest
- Trustworthy
- Responsible
- Caring
- Kind
- Thoughtful
- Open
- Brave
- Reliable
- Patient
- Generous
- Wise
- Open-minded
- Forgiving
- Humble
- Selfless
- Disciplined

- Loving
- Fun

Now, give examples of how your assets are manifested in your character.

It's important to do this. This is 'evidence' that we are not bad people and do have good parts to our personality. It's very easy for us to focus on the negative and the negative parts of our character can take over when we are drinking. However, in sobriety the better parts of ourselves will have a chance to shine. It's hard to be kind, patient and reliable when we are hung-over.

Activity – Reviewing assets and liabilities

1. Has anything on the list surprised you?
2. In what way has alcohol highlighted your character liabilities rather than your assets?

Explain and give examples.

What are my faulty beliefs?

We all have a belief system. For most of us this is unconscious, which means that we don't even recognise what we believe about ourselves and others, and nor do we understand the massive impact these subconscious beliefs have on our lives.

We form our beliefs about ourselves, the world and other people from our early experiences. The process of how we understand these experiences is how we create meaning and make sense of the world.

Beliefs are created by the *interpretations* we put on events. These thoughts and ideas that become our beliefs are mostly unquestioned. We accept them as facts. We treat our beliefs as realities, as immoveable truths. Because they emanate from inside us, they have great power over us. They govern our lives when we don't challenge them. We have both negative (limiting) and positive beliefs, and as you can guess, it's the negative beliefs that can cause the most damage. These negative beliefs can also be seen as our inner negative critic. It's that voice inside that says 'I'm not good enough', 'I can never do anything right', etc. These negative thoughts originate from our limiting beliefs.

This critical voice feeds on the limiting beliefs we have about ourselves.

Because this voice is so convincing, it ignores our strengths and assets and erodes our self-esteem. We often drink to drown out our negative critical voice.

Common limiting beliefs are:
- I'm stupid.
- I'm unattractive.
- I'm fat.
- I'm useless.
- I can't change.
- I'm not as good as other people.
- I'm not good enough.
- No one will love me.
- If people really knew me they wouldn't like me.
- I might get found out.
- If something goes right for me something always comes along and messes it up.
- Rich people are lucky – I'd be OK if I had money.
- Everyone else seems to know what they're doing.
- Life is hard.

They manifest themselves as a critical voice in this way:
- I'm so stupid. I forgot to ring a client back when I said I would.
- I'm useless. I might as well not bother – I never get picked.
- I'm a horrible person. No one likes me.
- I should be able to do …
- I must try harder to …
- I ought to be able to …

In order to overcome this internal critic and change our beliefs we have to do three things:
1. Discover what our limiting beliefs are
2. Challenge our limiting beliefs
3. Create new empowering beliefs.

Discovering our limiting beliefs

These limiting beliefs could be formed by experiences you had when you were young. I formed many limiting beliefs from experiences I had as a child and young adult. If I didn't get picked for something, or I felt rejected by friends, I always thought 'This is happening because I'm not good enough'. Eventually, that became my truth; I just felt I wasn't good enough and my behaviour kept reinforcing the belief. It became a self-fulfilling prophecy.

I can guarantee that as an alcoholic you will have more than your fair share of limiting and negative beliefs. Our messy, damaging, chaotic alcoholic behaviour would have provided very fertile ground for limiting beliefs to take root and grow. By the end of my drinking, my belief system was very negative; I believed that everything about me was negative. It wasn't until I got sober that I finally began to challenge these beliefs and to my amazement found out they weren't true! Gradually, I began to change them and guess what? When I began to change my beliefs my experience of life began to change.

Imagine who you'd be if you believed different things about yourself. Have you ever stopped to question what you believe about yourself? What happens is that we become what we think. So if we believe we aren't good enough, that no one likes us and we are losers, then our experience of life will reflect these thoughts.

Our beliefs are a *filter system*. Therefore your brain will filter out anything that doesn't fit with the beliefs you have created. It only accepts and captures information that fits your model of the world. It's like a fishing net.

If you are unhappy with the circumstances and consequences of your life, challenge your beliefs.

Let's discover what your limiting beliefs are.

Activity – Identifiying my limiting beliefs

Write down three things under each category.

1. <u>Beliefs about myself</u> (eg *'I'm a bad person'*, *'I don't deserve good things'*, *'I'm not attractive'*, *'I'm too old'*, *'If I was different, people would like me'*, *'I'm unlovable'*)

2. <u>Beliefs about the world</u> (eg *'Life is just not fair', 'Life is hard', 'Rich people are lucky', 'If I'm happy, something always comes along to spoil it', 'I'll never have enough of what I need', 'People are out to get me'*)

3. <u>Beliefs about relationships</u> (eg *'Men/Women can't be trusted', 'I always get let down or dumped', 'No one will ever love me', 'If my partner really knew me they would reject me', 'Men/Women only want one thing'*)

Challenging our limiting beliefs

Now that we have uncovered these limiting beliefs we need to challenge the power they have over us. You may be thinking 'Well, there's no point. I know they're true. They've always been true.' That thought is just another limiting belief. Put aside the negative voice for a moment and look more closely at where these beliefs come from.

Activity – Challenging my limiting beliefs

Look at the three beliefs you selected and ask yourself the following questions:

1. What event led me to form this belief?
2. Is this belief true?
3. Does this statement always hold up?
4. Will this thought be a positive factor in my recovery?

eg If your limiting belief was *'If I was different, people would like me'*, then your answers may look like this:

1. What event led me to form this belief?
   I can remember not being accepted by the 'cool' gang at school. I always thought that if I were better looking, cooler or just different, they would have liked me. I've thought that in nearly all of my relationships and friendships.

2. Is this belief true?

   Sometimes. I have some friends where I feel I can be myself and am liked for it. When I relax I find I don't really care what other people think but that doesn't happen very often. I guess I am hung up on what other people think rather than what I think. I would rather have two or three genuine friends than thirty 'fair-weather' friends. I often want to be liked by people I don't like or respect back. Maybe if I just focused on being myself I would find people I felt comfortable with, instead of trying to impress people, as this is a false way to live.

3. Does this statement always hold up?

   No, not really. It does when I think of all the people I felt rejected by but honestly I was just trying to impress them or seek their approval. They probably saw that. If I don't take a risk and let people see the real me then I don't give anyone a fair chance of liking me. Perhaps this is something I am creating myself? Without alcohol to hide behind I'm just going to have to be myself.

4. Is this limiting belief going to be a positive factor in my recovery?

   No, of course not. It keeps me trapped in a negative way of thinking about myself and when I feel negative I drink.

What we are looking to do is create cracks in our limiting beliefs. It's very easy to make our beliefs universal. Of course not everyone in the whole wide world is going to like you. And if you pretend to be someone you're not, people will sense that and reject that, but if you strive to be yourself you may find there are people out there who will respond and connect with you.

Apply the questions above to all of your limiting beliefs; see if you can create cracks in them. By doing this you will be moving away and quietening down that inner critical voice.

Creating new empowering beliefs

Now we have begun to dismantle these limiting beliefs we can actually create new empowering ones. We can continue to crush them by replacing them with something more positive.

Old belief	New belief
I'm a bad person.	I did some things I'm ashamed of in my alcoholism. That doesn't make me a bad person. Now I have the tools to change. I have many good parts to my character.
I don't deserve good things.	As I learn to love myself I can accept good things into my life.
Life is hard.	Sometimes life has been a struggle. Most of the time I have been my own worst enemy. If I work hard I can have a positive outcome.
People are out to get me.	Other people are too obsessed with themselves to worry about me! Often my own behaviour has caused consequences I don't like. When I behave differently I'll get different results.
Men/Women can't be trusted.	I've volunteered to be in really abusive relationships. I saw the warning signs and ignored them. I can make better choices now.

One of the problems with our limiting beliefs is that we just absorb these ridiculous universal thoughts and apply them to everything. Part of the work we are doing here is about making them 'right-sized'. Anyone who has a drink problem has done stuff they are ashamed of, but it doesn't make you a monster. Also, you must recognise how much your drink problem has affected your choices and behaviour. Although alcoholism turns us into unlikeable people, sobriety can change that. Every time your inner critic starts repeating a negative thought, challenge it and replace it with a more empowering one.

Who am I angry with and why?

In recovery circles you will hear the phrase 'resentments' a lot. Resentments are not unique to alcoholics; everyone gets resentments against other people; it's just part of being human. I would say that alcoholics however are the least equipped to deal with them. Resentments can cause us a lot of trouble. A resentment is when we feel anger towards someone for something we have perceived that they have done to us. We feel hurt, slighted or treated unjustly. When these feelings take root, they are toxic and poisonous to us.

Here are two telling statements about what resentment means:

1. Resentment: 'the number one offender', it literally means to re-feel. In reality it is the bearing of a grudge which tends to get worse each time you think of it.
2. *"Resentment is like drinking poison and wanting the other person to die."*

These two examples perfectly illustrate why it's completely unacceptable for us to continue harbouring resentments in our minds. It's not other people who suffer, it is us!

From *Why You Drink and How to Stop*:

Renting space in your head

Think about this. Who and what do you rent free space in your mind to? And what does that do to you? *No one inhabits your thoughts unless you invite them in.*

We allow other people's actions to dominate us by constantly going over in our minds conversations and situations that have troubled us. When we get caught up in worrying what other people think about us we are giving away our personal power. We do this when we are dissatisfied and are dominated by what other people may or may not have done to us. We just can't seem to let 'it' go. By going over old resentments and frustrations we are 'chewing' on them, often making them worse than they actually were.

If our mind is not free and we are chewing over negative feelings towards people then almost inevitably this will lead us to drink again. So in order to lay the foundations for successful, sustainable sobriety we must deal with these feelings.

Note that I used the word 'perceived' resentments. Some of our resentments may actually be down to perception rather than reality. It's

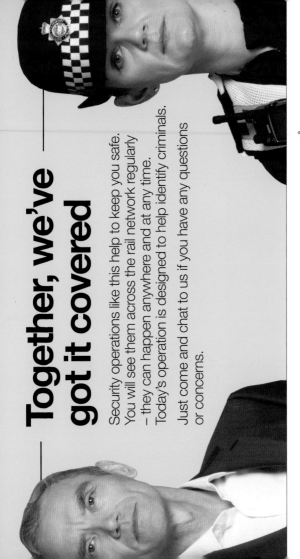

Together, we've got it covered

Security operations like this help to keep you safe. You will see them across the rail network regularly – they can happen anywhere and at any time. Today's operation is designed to help identify criminals.

Just come and chat to us if you have any questions or concerns.

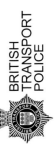

BRITISH TRANSPORT POLICE

For more information visit
btp.police.uk
PROJECT SERVATOR

Together we've got it covered

We use a range of security measures to help keep you safe. These might vary between operations, but here's a quick introduction to some of them.

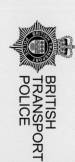

BRITISH TRANSPORT POLICE

Uniformed officers
Feel free to talk to our officers about today's operation. They will be happy to answer questions about what we are doing and why.

Search dogs
Our dogs are highly trained. They can search for things that could put others in danger.

Train patrols
You may see officers on board your train. They will be offering advice and looking for unattended belongings in an effort to reduce crime.

Plain clothed officers
They may be hard to spot, but they keep an eye out for people seeking to avoid our checks.

Searches
Officers have a range of powers they can use to stop and search individuals.

CCTV
Specially trained staff in our control rooms help us detect those intent on committing crime.

Other checks
We can also use other security measures that may not be visible.

Report anything that doesn't feel right
Tell a police officer or a member of staff
Call 0800 40 50 40
Text 61016

In an emergency call **999**

true that we may also have been harmed or abused by someone in our past. If this is the case then we need to look at how we have responded to those harms. *We may not have had a choice in what happened to us, but we do get to choose our response.* Has our response been an empowering one or one that caused us to continue the harm done to us?

Let's look more closely at who you are angry with and why. Answer the following questions as thoroughly as possible. Sample answers are given.

Activity – Resentment

1. Who rents space in my head and why?

   Make a list of people you are angry, irritated or frustrated with. Include anyone who just rents space in your head and causes you negative feelings. Next to each name give a brief explanation of how you feel towards this person and what you feel caused the situation.

   My boss – He is completely unreasonable and has no concept of my workload. He just piles on requests and never asks if it's OK. He also walks past me without acknowledging me.

   My ex-boyfriend – He was arrogant, rude and lazy. He never complimented me on my appearance and never did anything I wanted to do. I could never make him happy. Now he is in a new relationship and acts like he is Prince Charming. Why couldn't he have been that way for me?

2. What was my part in this?

   Once you have completed your list go back to the people on it and ask yourself 'What was my part in this'?

   My boss – I have never spoken up for myself or asked to meet with him and explain why sometimes it's challenging to get things done. I take it personally when he walks past me without saying hello when I also see him do this to other people, so I know it's not anything personal. Maybe he has a lot on his mind.

   My ex-boyfriend – Our relationship wasn't good from the start. There were plenty of 'red flags' that I just ignored because I wanted to have a 'boyfriend' so desperately. I never spoke up for myself or told him his behaviour was unacceptable. I taught him how he could treat me. I'm so afraid of being alone that I put up with this kind of behaviour.

3. What can I do differently?

Now we need to look at how we can choose to respond differently to the people who bother us.

My boss – I will make an appointment to address the issues I have with him. The rest of the stuff I'm just going to try and not take personally.

My ex-boyfriend – By doing this exercise I have clearly revealed a pattern of behaviour I just didn't want to see before. It's not that I'm just choosing the wrong men but I am setting myself up to fail before I even start. I know I have low self-esteem and now I can see how much it is impacting my romantic relationships. I need to get some help with this, as I don't want to keep repeating this pattern.

The purpose of this exercise is for us to gain freedom in our minds, to be free of the negative thoughts that we have towards people. When our minds are free then we are free to become a better version of ourselves.

It's very important to write these answers down. Allow yourself the time to go through the process and have the realisations you need to have.

What and who do I need to make peace with?

If you do this work thoroughly you may see that there are some relationships that you need to heal. This may mean making an apology, having a conversation or just spending time with someone you have been avoiding. Only you know what your relationships are like and what needs to be done. Don't let pride get in the way of your making a relationship right again. Pride can prevent us from showing humility, especially when we don't want to admit that we were wrong, or just apologise for our part in the situation.

Our pride can become a wall that we build around ourselves, that prevents the connection we need with other people. Courage and humility are required here. Start with one person and see what happens – you may be amazed at the results.

Where have I made assumptions and not communicated my needs?

It was very revealing to me when I saw that I was actually responsible for some of the dysfunction in my relationships. I often expected people to read my mind and automatically know what I wanted or needed. When they didn't, I blamed them. I was rarely honest about my feelings, so never communicated my needs to people or set proper boundaries. Then I would get upset and resentful when I felt my needs were ignored.

We need to stop expecting people to be mind readers and learn to articulate our needs.

Activity – Assumptions and needs

Identify where in your relationships you have made assumptions or not communicated your needs, resulting in hurt or confusion.

1. What assumptions have I made in my friendships/relationships? (eg *I pretend everything is OK when it's not because I expect them to know I'm upset. I'm angry and hurt when they don't realise that I am.*)
2. What usually happens when I don't communicate my needs to people? (*I'm hurt and angry with them so then I want to punish them for hurting me.*)
3. What could you do differently? (*I could tell my friends that I'm not doing well instead of smiling and nodding. I could swallow my pride and let them help me.*)

Your answers will reveal to you the changes you need to make in your communication with people. This is really a skill that we have never learnt to use properly. Like all skills, it takes practice. Start with small steps, pay attention to how you feel and practise.

What messes do I need to clean up?

If you have an alcohol problem then the chances are that you have created some 'messes' in your life: relationships that have gone sour for no clear reason; groups we dropped because we couldn't cope; situations at work that we didn't deal with because we were hung-over; neighbours we have upset because of our thoughtlessness.

As part of our recovery we will feel better about ourselves if we can begin to clear up some of these 'messes'.

Activity – Messes

Start a list of 'messes' that you want to clean up. After you've created your list, write down what it is you need to do. Is it apologise, pay back some money, explain the situation? It's best to keep it as simple as possible. Remember not to criticise or blame the other person – just stick to your own side of the street.

Dealing with my relationships

Improving our relationships with other people is a key part of our recovery. Put simply, we *need* other people. We *need* connection and we *need* belonging, they are essential to our well-being. Loneliness is the enemy of the alcoholic. Most of us could use help in improving our relationships. This will often take time and a lot of patience on our part. We can start by looking at our relationships with our family members. Family dynamics are often complex; sometimes we have been stuck in a pattern of behaviour for decades. Looking more closely at these relationships is the first step towards changing how we interact with family members.

Activity – Relationship with parents

Describe your relationship with your parents.

1. What did you learn from your parents? eg What did they teach you about love, anger, drinking?
2. What issues of their own were they dealing with?
3. What do you need to forgive them for?

These are powerful questions because our parental relationships have a huge impact on our lives.

As I wrote in *Why You Drink and How to Stop*:

Whether we had a good or bad experience growing up, our parents have a profound and long lasting impact on our lives, often without our realising. We will always be their child, no matter how old we are, and our task is to become independent of them: free of their baggage, which we inadvertently picked up.

Even if your parents were absent, you will still have to deal with your experience of not being parented adequately. Co-dependency can often occur in adult and child relationships, and can continue into the child's adult life.

Without realising it, parents can convey strong messages: that the child needs to please the parents in order to receive their love, or that the child exists to provide the parent with the love they never received. This can be when the seeds of co-dependency are planted. We can grow into adults who are never free of the unhealthy chains that bind us to our parents' approval. Often, our parents don't realise what they are doing, and may never recognise their behaviour, so we have to be responsible for 'unchaining' ourselves.

The words *mother* and *father* are two of the most powerful words we have in our vocabulary, and are usually the first words we learn. They are powerful because of the *meanings* we attach to them. The word 'mother' in our culture generally means: love, comfort, support, tenderness, safety, gentleness, caring, etc. The word 'father' in our culture generally means: discipline, order, authority, power, fun, guidance, leader, etc. When you take these words away from the person, all you have left is a person who is trying to do the best they can, however inadequate that may actually be.

The words 'Mum' and 'Dad' are powerful because of these meanings; we project onto them an image of perfection. No one can live up to what the word suggests. Like you, mums and dads are works in progress.

So, one of the keys to freedom is to let go of your parents, and what they did and didn't do to you. They are just people after all. Have a relationship with them, but stop getting angry or frustrated with them. Stop blaming them. You only keep yourself chained if you don't.

Now here's the deal: your parents are human beings too and they were doing the best they could with the tools they had available. All their behaviour was about them, and not you. This is very important. The way your parents behaved didn't have anything to do with their loving you or not loving you.

This stuff can be very complicated, not to mention painful, so I'll try and make it as simple as possible. At some point, we do have to 'let go' of our parents. You may have had an absent or abusive parent – sexually, mentally, emotionally or physically – or an inadequate parent. You may have had a parent who wasn't fully 'present' because they were so wrapped up in themselves. You may have had a parent who couldn't express love. It's important that you know that *these were their failings, not yours*!

Abuse of any kind, especially by a parent, is a terrible thing. However, it wasn't your fault, and it certainly wasn't because you weren't good enough. However, this is the interpretation we come to, because when we are children we take everything personally. In fact, as adults we also take everything personally. We interpret the world personally. We interpret everyone else's behaviour to mean something personal, *especially* that of our parents. Knowing this is enormously freeing. Our parents were caught up in their own 'stuff', which sometimes had an impact on you.

So now it's time to see your parents as the flawed human beings they are. There's nothing bad about that; maybe they worked on themselves, maybe they didn't. Whatever their failings were, don't take responsibility for them. They're not yours. Put them down and experience what it's like to be free from that baggage.

We pick up lots of unwanted stuff from our parents: guilt, shame, feelings of not being good enough and so on. Now is the time to recognise this: *'uncover, discover, discard'*.

Activity – Improving relationship with parents

What can you do to improve your relationship with your parents? Remember, it's not about your parents changing, it's about *you* changing. It might be something like having better boundaries (we look more closely at how to create boundaries in the next section) with your parents, or being more open with them. It's a process.

The purpose of this exercise is to take the first step in that process.

You can also apply the same questions to sibling relationships.

Romantic relationships

Let's move on to looking at romantic relationships. I have yet to meet an alcoholic who didn't have trouble in that area.

From *Why You Drink and How to Stop*:

I 'engineered' all of my relationships. I was controlling and manipulative. Some of the men I had relationships with I cared for, but the truth was that they were never based on love. They were based on fear. Fear of:
- Loneliness
- Not being loved

- Being 'left on the shelf'.

And once *in* the relationship, the fear was of:

- Not being good enough
- Being rejected
- Having them discover who I really was.

Plain old fear. Lots of it.

I found there were plenty of emotionally messed up men, who were more than happy to engage in this warped dance. I used sex to get love, and attracted men who used love to get sex. It's a game that men and women have been playing since time began.

Relationships in recovery can be equally hazardous, because without the security blanket of alcohol we are laid bare. We are exposed and we are most definitely frightened as hell. Romantic relationships key into our deepest fears of not being worthy of love. We are frightened of the other person getting too close, seeing who we really are and rejecting us, thus confirming what we believed in the first place – a faulty belief, by the way. So from the start we are unconsciously pushing the other person away and acting on this faulty belief and, in this way, we create this as our experience again and again. And thus the faulty belief is reinforced.

It's as though we have completely bought the fairytale, and believe true love will solve all our problems, if only we could find it. All love stories end when the couple fall in love and kiss. This is the implied solution. Everything will be perfect now because love conquers all. But this is actually when the hard work really starts, because in reality 'our true love' is an imperfect human being who has their own emotional baggage, just as we do.

In order to attract into our lives the relationships we want, or to improve the relationship we are in, it will benefit us hugely to look at our patterns and mistakes in romantic relationships. Once we have discovered our negative patterns in relationships, we can then find a way to be free of the unhealthy behaviour.

Activity – Romantic relationships

Answer the following questions as honestly and in as much detail as you can.

1. How did alcohol affect your relationship?
   (Were your relationships based on drinking? What were your dates like – did they always involve alcohol? Were you drunk when you had sex for the first time with someone? How did your relationships end? Did alcohol fuel conflict in your relationships?)
2. Have your relationships been based on love or fear?
   (When we are insecure and needy, our relationships tend to be based on fear. We are frightened we are going to be 'left behind', or that no one will ever love us. The fear of being alone is the motivator for staying in an abusive and dysfunctional relationship – I speak from experience here. What have you put up with because you were frightened? Where have you compromised your values or beliefs?)
3. How do you move the 'goal posts'?
   (Moving the 'goal posts' is when we have set standards we believe we won't compromise, but when faced with the possibility of losing romantic love, we do compromise those standards. How have you done this? Are there things you promised you would never do or say that you have (and then regretted) in order to keep a partner? What have been the consequences?)
4. How did you learn about relationships? Who were your teachers?
   (We are taught about 'love' primarily from our family relationships. Subconsciously we absorb these implicit messages into our own belief systems. What were your parents', grandparents', aunts' and uncles' relationships like? Were they good roles models, or the opposite? Did you look at any of these relationships and promise yourself you would be different?)

Recognising co-dependency

In *Why You Drink and How to Stop* I wrote:

In essence, co-dependents manage their feelings, identity and self-worth by trying to manage other people. Co-dependency is ultimately about controlling the environment around them so that they can control their own inner turmoil.

There are two types of co-dependency:

TYPE I

The co-dependent will expend an enormous amount of energy attempting to control people in their environment. They will lie, manipulate, blame and control others around them into being or doing what the co-dependent wants them to be or do. The motivation for this behaviour is that the co-dependent believes they will then be happy (safe), and the people around them will be happy too (they just don't know it yet!).

TYPE II

The other way co-dependency can be expressed is when the co-dependent has no sense of 'self' and becomes whatever they believe others want them to be. They are chameleons, forever changing their outsides to suit who they are with. They lose themselves, and can make no decision or choice by their own volition. It is always to suit the person they are with – parent, friend or lover. They constantly feel desperate because they never feel good enough. They feel like failures because no matter how hard they try to be what they believe their significant other wants them to be, they always fail. Again, the motivation for this behaviour is that this type of co-dependent believes they will finally be happy or safe, once they have pleased or satisfied the people around them. They repeat this over and over, trying harder and harder each time.

Recognising and recovering from our co-dependency is essential to successful, sustainable sobriety. Why? Because the emotional intensity of a relationship can leave us vulnerable and un-anchored. Because if we blindly walk into another relationship based on past patterns we are setting ourselves up for pain and heartbreak. Until we develop robust methods to deal with these unpleasant feelings, then the chances of our defaulting to our natural coping strategy, intoxication, will be high.

This is why we must look at these patterns. Once we learn these things about ourselves we are empowered to overcome them.

Activity – Co-dependency

1. Have you tried to control loved ones through manipulation, bullying or having a 'hidden agenda'?
2. How do you feel when people don't do what you want them to do? (Do you feel resentful, hurt, frustrated, angry? What happens next?)
3. Do you lose yourself in relationships? (Do you 'become' whatever you feel the other person wants you to be? Do you 'like' what they 'like'? Do you have trouble identifying your own feelings?)
4. Describe your pattern in a romantic relationship. (How do your relationships start? How do they end? Do you have gaps in your relationships, or does one blend into another?)

With the information you have discovered from these answers you will have an idea of what changes you need to make and where you need to start. It is also important to have a good idea of what our ideal relationship would look like. This was something I'd never really given much thought to. Because I didn't know what a healthy functioning relationship looked like, I kept settling for less than I deserved.

Activity – Relationship ideal

What is your relationship ideal?

1. How would you treat each other?
2. How would you resolve conflict?
3. What do you need in a relationship?

By getting a clear idea of what you want, you have a better chance of recognising it when it comes your way.

Friendships

Our peer relationships are another area that we can work on, especially if many of our friendships are based on drinking. We are not looking to disregard friendships just because we don't drink any more; rather we want to identify which friendships have a positive impact in our lives and which ones don't. Whilst drinking, my friendships were often toxic and uncomfortable. I didn't really know how to be a 'good friend'. I was often manipulative and dishonest in my friendships, which doesn't allow for a climate of trust.

In the same that way we looked at our relationships, we are also going to look more closely at our friendship patterns.

Activity – Friendships

1. Do you have a pattern with friendships? What is it?
    (Do you have intense short-term friendships? Have you maintained friendships from the past? Do you make friends easily?)
2. Who do you consider your close friends? What defines your relationship?
    (How much is drinking part of your relationship? Do you do other things together that don't involve alcohol?)
3. Do you trust people easily?
4. How do you react if someone lets you down?
    (Have you felt resentful towards friends? How does that affect your relationship?)
5. Does your peer group support and encourage you, or does it limit you?
6. How have your friends reacted to your stopping drinking?
    (This is very revealing and will help you determine who is a good friend and who is maybe a 'fair-weather' friend. Drinkers really

don't like it when other drinkers quit and they may exert a lot of
pressure on you to drink again. A true friend will support you in
what you are trying to do.)

You can also apply these questions to any colleagues and working
relationships you have. We are looking for patterns of behaviour.
When we spot a pattern, we can learn something about ourselves and
make changes if the consequences of the pattern are not pleasing to
us. There were many things I had to change in my interactions with
family, friends and colleagues. I had lots of destructive patterns of
behaviour, most of them based on fear and insecurity, that caused
me to behave in ways that weren't authentic or congruent. Now, all
of my relationships are more honest and therefore more meaningful.
When we apply this work to ourselves, the fear diminishes, and we
can forgive ourselves and become likeable people.

Getting on with people, dealing with conflict, and dealing with the
difficulties that sometimes present themselves in relationships is another
skill that can be learnt. We can learn to say 'no', we can learn to have
boundaries. We can remove 'toxic' people from our lives. In Section 3 I
will go over the ways you can improve all your relationships by developing and applying these skills.

The section we have just been through can be tough going. If you
have answered the questions as honestly and thoroughly as possible, then
you have probably learnt a lot about yourself and discovered a lot of the
underlying causes of your drinking. Hopefully, you have revealed the
feelings and emotions that motivated your need to anaesthetise yourself.
Emotional pain has to be treated. If we are scared, ashamed, embarrassed,
lonely or angry then at some point we have to treat those feelings. The
choice we have is to carry on as we were, with the same results, or to try
a different way of living.

Activity – Self-understanding

What have you learnt about yourself through doing this work?

Section 3

Freedom

BY NOW YOU will have learnt that getting sober is not as straight-forward as putting down the drink and resolving never to drink again. A bit of work is required, but luckily the work we put into getting sober is far easier than the work we put into maintaining our drink problem. As I highlighted in my first book, *Why You Drink and How to Stop*, the reason we drink the way we do is that it helps us cope with feelings and emotions that we have no other method of coping with. By completing Sections 1 and 2, you have revealed to yourself why you drink the way you do. Uncovering the destructive emotional patterns that drive our drinking means that we now have the ability to effect change. We can't solve this problem until we understand what the problem *actually is*. It was never external circumstances but internal conditions.

Section 3 is going to look at how you can change those patterns, feel differently and get control of your life again.

This section is split into two parts: we are going to look at 'sober tools' that can be applied to your life right now, and 'sober goals' that you are working towards.

We looked at how you can begin to deal with resentments and limiting beliefs in Section 2. In this section we are going to look at how we can respond to the world differently and so improve our relationships. When we uncovered the resentments and difficulties in our relationships, we identified where we could begin to make those relationships healthy again. But how do we prevent problems from starting in the first place?

How can we feel comfortable dealing with people in the workplace and in personal relationships? One of the most important and effective things we can do is to have boundaries and learn to say 'no'.

Learning to say 'no'

When I was drinking I was the worst 'people pleaser'. I was so scared you wouldn't like me that I would do whatever I could to please you. Because I believed I would then have your approval (whoever you were) and everything would be OK. That was my formula for life. Be liked, no matter what.

My self-esteem and entire sense of wellbeing became based on other people's approval. So I never said 'no'. Instead, I said 'yes' and often regretted it. I'd often have to back-pedal out of my 'yes's because I rarely meant them. Or I'd just lie, or not show up, or avoid you, or manufacture elaborate reasons that sadly, unfortunately, and regrettably I couldn't do what I had so fervently agreed to just a matter of days (or hours) earlier.

Saying yes when I didn't mean it made me a liar, a manipulator, a false friend, a time waster, an idiot and unreliable. You know the sort of person I mean.

I was also very easily manipulated, because it was so apparent that my desire for you to like me was so much bigger than my desire to like myself.

When I got sober I soon realised that saying 'yes' when I didn't mean it caused me all sorts of problems and quandaries. I began to see that if I continued behaving this way, it would become so uncomfortable that I'd drink again. So I had to learn to say 'no'. My 'yes' had to mean 'yes', and my 'no' had to mean 'no'.

The first thing I learnt was that I had to learn to like myself. That what I thought of myself was actually far more important than what other people thought of me. In many ways, by doing the work laid out in this book, you are taking the first steps towards liking yourself again, because you are taking responsibility for the direction of your life.

So, I had to learn to say 'no', because when I said 'yes' and didn't mean it, I liked myself less. I became uncomfortable in my own skin and that is a dangerous situation for an alcoholic to be in. I had to take a deep breath and say 'No, thank you.'

When I did this, I learnt that *your* feelings were *your* responsibility, and *my* feelings were *mine*.

That if you were upset by my 'no' although I had said it politely, how you felt about it wasn't my responsibility. This revolutionised my life.

Firstly, I began to like myself more. By uttering this one small word honestly and where necessary, I began to become a person of integrity. I became reliable, I showed up when I said I would, I did what I had agreed to do and I meant what I said. You could trust me.

Now, after fifteen years, it's easy, but at the time it was the hardest thing I'd ever done. I know I'm not alone. Lots of people get sober and discover there's a whole bunch of life skills they missed out on developing. Staying sober isn't just staying away from alcohol. It's learning a whole new way of living in the world. And learning to say 'no' can be one of the most lifesaving skills. Because one of the best things about getting sober is all the wonderful things you can say 'yes' too.

So let's look a little more closely at how exactly we can learn this small but important skill.

'No' is such a little word but it has powerful implications. Before I get into how to say 'no', I need you to understand why we are so afraid of actually using this small but powerful word.

The main reason is that we are scared of what other people will think about us.

We are also scared of:
- Not being liked
- Disappointing someone
- Being wrong
- Making a mistake
- Being rejected
- Potential conflict
- Feeling uncomfortable or others feeling uncomfortable
- Hurting someone's feelings
- Causing upset.

The main reason we are scared of saying 'no' is that we misguidedly believe that we are responsible for how other people feel. So instead of saying 'no' when we need to, we become liars. You probably consider yourself to be a 'good' person, an honest person even, so it may come as a shock to you that when you say 'yes' and don't mean it, you are actually a liar. Oh yes, you're also a thief. A liar and a thief.

That's probably a shock to you, right? You've probably never 'stolen' anything in your life and you are sitting there reading this feeling very outraged at the mere suggestion. Well, here's the thing: if you lie and say 'yes' when you mean 'no', you could very well be stealing someone's learning and growth opportunity from them.

Here's why: let's say I need to move house this weekend and I'm a pretty disorganised person. My life is always a bit crazy and I'm pretty good at coercing people into doing what I want them to do. It's always worked for me, so why change?

I come to you with a look of tragedy on my face, and my sob story of how I desperately need help moving this weekend. You look at me and see my furrowed brow, hear the plaintive cries that signal my distress, and inside you're panicking.

Because the last thing you ever want to do is hurt someone's feelings. But you have plans this weekend and you absolutely cannot help me. A feeling of dread washes over you. The conversation goes like this:

'[Insert your name here], I really, really need your help. Everyone's let me down. I don't know what I'm going to do. I have to move but I have no one to help me. Please, please can you spare some time to just give me a hand?'

And you reply, 'Sure, absolutely. Of course I can help. Don't worry.'

And your internal voice is going, 'Noooooooo! Why did you ever agree to that?'

All week, every time you think of the weekend, you get that sinking feeling in your stomach. You run all these scenarios in your head: maybe if I get there really early, maybe I can help for a bit then sneak off, maybe …

The more you think about it, the worse you feel. Then you start getting very annoyed. How come you always get landed with this stuff? How come you are always the person helping others out?

Then Friday night comes around and the absolute last thing you want to do is help this person move at the weekend. You are resentful, mad and full of self-pity. So you text them: 'I'm so sorry. I'm sick, been in bed all day. No way I can help tomorrow. So sorry to let you down.' And relief floods your body, because you have found a way of getting out of doing something you really never wanted to do in the first place.

However, there is a sting, because you've lied. You are a liar.

But you justify it, rationalise it: it's only a *white* lie, it's not a big one. Besides, you had to lie, you were forced to. Then you feel a little better. Does this sound familiar? Have you ever done anything like that?

I used to do that stuff all the time. I was always agreeing to do things with people but freaking out inside. My insides and my outsides didn't match. I would think one thing but *do or say another.* Can you see that when we act like this it makes us feel very uncomfortable, and if we stay feeling this way for long enough we will use booze to deal with the feelings?

So, here's the thing. The person who needed to move, are they in a quandary? Sure they are. They have been let down at the last minute. They have a mess to figure out.

But what if you and everyone else they had asked that week had been honest. What if you had said, 'No, I'm sorry. I have plans that I can't change.' Would that person have walked away upset? Sure they would.

But then maybe, just maybe, they would have started thinking, 'This always happens to me. I always leave everything to the last minute. I'm always having to run around and sell my sob story to try to get people to do what I want them to. I'm sick of this. I need to get my act together. I need to organise and plan my life better.'

Bingo. Right there, a learning and growth opportunity has arisen.

Maybe they needed this uncomfortable situation in order to learn from it. It is actually pain and discomfort that motivate us to change. *If you try to save me from those feelings, then you also steal from me the things that motivate me to change.*

Our greatest learning and growth opportunities often come from the messes we make in our lives.

Saying 'no' takes practice. It feels scary and hard to start with. If you had said 'no' right at the beginning to your friend, would they have walked away upset? Yes, probably.

Now pay very close attention, because the next bit is important. Did you cause that upset? No, you didn't.

If you politely and kindly say 'no', how the other person feels about that is neither your business nor your responsibility. You are not responsible for how other people feel. You are only responsible for how you feel.

Now, if you had said to your friend, 'Get lost, you creep. I wouldn't help you if you were the last person on earth', would you have had a part in upsetting them? Of course. You were mean and rude, and that tends to upset people. But do you see the difference?

People may be disappointed, hurt, angry or upset if you say 'no' to what they ask. But as long as you say it politely, there isn't anything you can do about their feelings. Manipulative people in particular will communicate their disappointed feelings to you, because these are the tools they use to get people to do what they want. Think about that.

It's our fear of how other people are going to feel, and our faulty belief that we are responsible for these feelings, that gets us into situations we don't want to be in.

There are only so many things we can agree to do; there are only so many hours in the day. We need to say 'no' sometimes to bring balance into our lives. But more importantly, other people need to experience what it's like to have a 'no' sometimes. Don't steal that learning opportunity from them.

There is a wonderful phrase (I think it's from Al-Anon) that sums this all up beautifully:

"Say what you mean, mean what you say and don't say it mean."

Trust me, applying that simple rule to your life will transform it. Because when you say 'yes' you will mean it. People know I'm going to show up and do stuff; they know my 'yes' means 'yes' and my 'no' means 'no'.

It can feel uncomfortable practising this at first. Naturally, we don't want other people to be upset or disappointed, as compassionate human beings we would like to avoid that if we can. So we may feel a brief 'after-burn' when we see that someone else is disappointed. But we must be clear: we aren't responsible for other people's feelings. It is not our job to rescue others from uncomfortable emotions just because we can't bear to witness them. We can't please everyone, it's impossible.

We cause more upset when we say 'yes' and don't mean it, then later on have to wriggle our way out of what we agreed to do. This causes frustration and consternation. We are unreliable, people can't trust us, they don't know when we are going to let them down. Then our behaviour causes upset. This is the part that needs to change.

I can promise you that this gets easier and easier. There are lots of things I can say 'yes' to, but I don't over-schedule myself anymore. I will help you move if I'm able to. And if I can't, I'll let you know right away so that you can plan accordingly.

The most important thing now is *how I feel about myself.* I have no control over others. I can't move mountains just because I think it will make you feel better. I am no longer chained by the good or bad opinion of others. How I feel about myself is the only thing I have full control over.

I would suggest starting this new behaviour with small steps and with people you are at least semi-comfortable with. It really does get easier with practice but it is natural to feel nervous or even frightened when you think about saying 'no' to someone. This is perfectly natural; I felt exactly the same way. If you are a chronic people pleaser like I was, this can seem daunting at first, but focus on how you are going to feel afterwards. By saying 'no', you will have freed your mind from all that worry and concern you create when saying 'yes' and not meaning it. Imagine how free you will feel. After you say 'no' for the first time, pay attention to the feelings and emotions swirling around inside you – it might be useful to write them down. Remember that by doing this you have taken a massive step towards becoming responsible for your feelings instead of being at the mercy of them. You have removed one more reason for why you drink.

How to have boundaries in your life

I had no idea what boundaries were until I got sober. I had no idea that I could protect my personal space and keep myself safe. I was so used to doing what I thought everyone else wanted that I would continuously put myself in risky and abusive situations. So setting boundaries was one more life lesson I had to learn. Boundaries are *our* responsibility; we can't expect other people to protect them for us. Other people may invade or run over our boundaries and it is our job to put the boundary back in place. Saying 'no' is a boundary; it puts a limit on what we can do and what we can't.

I also thought that there were certain people I couldn't have boundaries with, such as family members. Actually, you can. I had a particularly difficult relationship with one family member. I was never able to say 'no' and always felt frustrated and resentful towards them. When I learnt to set boundaries I realised that I could only do what I felt capable of doing. If people were hurt or offended by that, then I just had to let them be hurt and offended as I wasn't responsible for their feelings. As I began to assert my boundaries with family in the shape of 'No, I can't spend all weekend with you but I can meet you for lunch next Wednesday', I found that they adjusted. I accepted that they wanted to see me (compromise) but it was going to be on my terms. When they pushed (and they will) I just politely and firmly repeated my boundary. I didn't get angry. I expected them to challenge my boundary and was prepared. Over time this got easier and easier. We allow others to violate our boundaries in many different ways. Here are some examples:

- Not being able to say 'no'
- Violating personal values or beliefs in order to please others
- When giving to others causes you to suffer
- Letting other people make decisions for you and not speaking up when we don't like them
- Not standing up for yourself because you're scared you will offend someone
- Expecting others to know what your needs are and fulfill them automatically
- Expecting someone will take care of you and not helping yourself when you can
- Agreeing with others because it's easier
- Never letting your real feelings show.

These are just some of the ways we give permission for other people to abuse us. Developing healthy boundaries takes time and practice. But if we begin to implement them into all areas of our lives, we will notice that how we feel changes. Having boundaries is a way for us to feel in control of our feelings rather than at the mercy of others.

Let's go over what *healthy boundaries* look like. These are the boundaries we need to adopt and implement in our lives.

- Saying 'yes' when you mean it
- Saying 'no' when you mean it
- Not over explaining answers
- Not giving unnecessary explanations
- Understanding that you are responsible for your own feelings
- Identifying the causes of your feelings
- Responding with appropriate feelings to appropriate events
- Resisting the urge to 'rescue' others
- Being able to ask for help
- Making time for self-care and self-love
- Prioritising what is important to you
- Being with people you choose to be with
- Gracefully removing toxic relationships from your life
- Saving yourself.

Developing boundaries is a process; it will take time. You will make mistakes. That's OK. Be gentle with yourself and move forward at your own pace. These tools will help you to build a robust defence against drinking again.

Dealing with toxic people

Most alcoholics have some very dysfunctional and difficult people in their lives. Some of these people are so 'toxic' they cause us distress and hurt every time we interact with them. As adults we don't have to put up with this. Even if these people are family members, we don't have to put up with abusive, destructive or toxic behaviour.

Dealing with toxic people is just one of those things you have to learn to do in recovery. I will admit it can be challenging sometimes; we can't remove people but have to settle at keeping them at arm's length.

With family members that we can't refuse to see, we can have very, very strong boundaries and only do what is comfortable for us. It may be the case that we have been manipulated by this person and they will exert a lot of pressure on us, which is another reason why boundaries are so important.

Toxic people tend to be resistant to change or to any kind of self-reflection; they are adamant that others have the problem and need to change instead. They generate drama and misery wherever they go and are incapable of seeing themselves as the cause of it. They are capable of very nasty and vindictive behaviour; they inflict pain as a form of punishment. They are nearly always negative.

In contrast, we can all have toxic 'moments' and we have probably indulged in some really toxic behaviour when drinking. We all behave badly sometimes but we are also capable of acknowledging this, owning it, making amends and changing.

It's really rather simple: everybody has their own rubbish. Some people are working on it; others are not. Pay attention and you will be able to spot the difference. The people who do not work on themselves are choosing to remain toxic.

I really believe that if there is someone in our lives who is abusive, and inflicting pain, then, for our own sakes, we have to remove them from our lives. If this is a family member, this will be an opportunity for you to practise your boundaries. Remember that you are not responsible for how they feel; you are only responsible for your own feelings. Yes, they may be offended if you distance yourself from them but this is a consequence of their actions. Allow them their consequences.

I also think that the more we work on ourselves, the fewer toxic people we attract into our experience, and this also helps. Maybe some of these people will change and we can invite them back into our lives, but sometimes they don't. What often happens when we remove toxic people from our lives is that we create space for someone wonderful to come in.

The important thing to know here is that despite the toxic relationships we have engaged in, we must keep our hearts open. We don't want to build a wall around ourselves and exclude people from our lives for fear of being hurt. Today, I assume people have good intentions, but if they show me otherwise then I set up boundaries. I occasionally come across a toxic person but mostly I meet really wonderful people. We need genuine human connection and must ensure we always leave a path open for that.

I passionately believe that we are responsible for the experience we wish to have; therefore we have to take responsibility for whom we invite into that experience. If we can balance this and keep our hearts open, then we are well on our way to becoming healthy functioning human beings.

Activity – Toxic people

1. Make a list of the toxic people in your life.
2. What boundaries can you put in place now to deal with the toxic people you have listed?

How to deal with feelings more effectively

We have just explored a practical strategy that will change your life and help you manage how you feel. For successful, sustainable sobriety it is also essential for us to manage our feelings appropriately. One of the most effective ways of doing this is to write them down. As alcoholics we are often unsure where our feelings originate from or what they are linked to. We are a big cauldron of emotions (mostly negative) that swirl around inside us. Because we are so disconnected from ourselves, and have numbed our feelings for so long, one of our tasks in recovery is to begin to connect once again with how we feel. This may mean wading through a backlog of feelings that have not been processed or dealt with in a healthy manner.

Activity – Identifying, analysing and challenging your feelings

1. To try to make sense of and find a path through your feelings, start writing them down every day. Where you can, see if you can connect them to an event.

eg *'I felt frightened and anxious when my boss told me he wanted to meet with me later.'*

There are many reasons why you might feel anxious or frightened about this event, but what I find is that our feelings, particularly fear, quickly get out of control.

2. Once you have identified a feeling, drill down to see what is underneath it.

   eg *'I'm frightened that I will lose my job. I'm frightened that my partner will leave me if I don't have a job. I'm frightened of being abandoned and alone. I'm frightened that I will never be loved.'*

   This is an example of my old thinking. Fear always felt overwhelming to me and I discovered it was because it was always linked to something deeper.

3. Once you have identified your true feelings, try challenging them. Ask yourself if this is true.

You may find that when you examine your feelings more closely and unpack them (much as we did with limiting beliefs) they begin to lose their power over you. If you do this exercise regularly, you will find in time that it becomes a natural response and you will be able to do it automatically at the time of the event. This skill will enable you to have mastery over your emotional life.

Letting go of 'perfect'

This section could be written really briefly. Here's the gist of it: 'You're not perfect. Get over it.' If only it were that simple, right?

Unfortunately, the disease of perfectionism is much more insidious than that; in fact it's a killer. Perfectionism will take you right back to the bottle if you let it.

But where does it come from?

Perfectionism is driven by an internal fear that we are not good enough. It is really an outward manifestation of emotional unmanageability. People who are a slave to perfectionism are trying to manage their 'insides' by ensuring their 'outsides' are perfect. Nothing is ever good enough for them; it's never quite right, no matter how hard they work. Perfection is always just out of their grasp. It taunts them with its promise that 'all will be well' once you have got 'it' perfect.

Alcoholics can be very prone to this behaviour. We reach for perfection, fail to achieve it, then drown our feelings of failure in alcohol. It's a vicious cycle.

Even if we achieve perfection in some aspect of our lives, it is unsustainable. Someone usually comes along and spoils it. If we keep trying to make our outside world perfect in order to feel happy or satisfied, then we will never be able to achieve sustainable happiness.

Why? Because the outside world is beyond our control. No matter how much effort we exert, we simply can't control others or what they do. They come along and mess up our perfect homes, plans, parties, holidays, events and so on. They don't do things the way we want them done – how they clearly should be done! – for everything to be 'perfect'. We feel frustrated and unhappy because things are not perfect. But perfection is an illusion.

We weren't designed to be perfect, we were made to be messy because that is how we learn. Children are the best example of this. They don't care if their clothes or room are a mess, or that they didn't colour in within the lines; their satisfaction comes from engaging with what's in front of them and embracing the experience. As adults we forget that the real joy lies in the experience and all it encompasses, not in whether it was done the 'right' way. When we are trying to be perfect we are actually letting that negative voice in our head take over.

Letting go of perfectionism can be a life changing and liberating experience. When we let go of it we are able to live in the moment, and accept what comes our way with grace and gratitude. When we are a slave to perfectionism we miss so much good stuff, like opportunities to grow and connect with people.

I remember an occasion when I was in the grasp of perfectionism. I attended a party a friend of mine had organised. When I arrived (on time), I discovered that nothing had really been organised properly. The decorations were only half up, the food wasn't ready, the music hadn't been organised. I was horrified. I remember thinking, 'How could the host possibly let this happen? I would feel so ashamed.' But then I noticed something: she was standing in the middle of it all radiating serenity and joy as people arrived. She calmly handed out tasks and guests happily completed the preparations. I was roped into sorting out the music with a guest I'd never met before. We had an absolute blast organising the playlist, laughing over each other's musical tastes and arguing for songs we loved. I looked around and saw the same thing was happening everywhere. Within minutes the party was pulled together and everyone had a fantastic time, including the host. It really stopped me in my tracks. I would have lost sleep over ensuring everything was perfect. I would have been stressed by the time everyone arrived and I wouldn't have really enjoyed the party because I would have been fretting over things going wrong. I would only have been relieved once everyone was leaving.

But what would that have achieved? That experience was for me the beginning of letting go of my perfectionism and embracing mess as something joyous. It takes practice. The thought of not being perfect used to induce anxiety in me and I had to learn how to let go of it. But bit by bit I did. And believe me, life is so much richer and more rewarding when you're not trying to be perfect.

Mistakes are the juice of life

By letting go of perfectionism I was able to see that messes and mistakes are actually the juice of life. That they gave me opportunities to grow and learn. As long as we take the opportunity to grow and learn from our mistakes, there is actually great freedom and liberation in making mistakes. Mistakes have a massive potential to stimulate spiritual and emotional growth.

The gifts that mistakes can bring into your life should not be underestimated.

I would even go as far as to say that making mistakes is a vital process in our lives; without them we wouldn't be able to succeed. Does that sound crazy?

Think about a young child again: every single part of their learning and growth comes from making mistakes! Learning to walk, for instance. They fall over, bump into things, even hurt themselves. They get it wrong a lot, before they get it right.

We never ever look at them and say, 'Well, maybe she's just not a walker.' We know that every time they fall over they learn something vital.

Making mistakes is just part of our learning process. But something happens when we become adults: that permission we had as children to mess up disappears and we develop a faulty belief that we are not allowed to mess up. That it's wrong to mess up, and that mistakes are bad. Because we misunderstand the purpose of mistakes, we are filled with guilt and shame and these feelings block the learning and the growth that can come from making the mistake. Mistakes are really just gifts in terrible packaging. If we don't see the 'gift' then we are doomed to repeat the same mistake over and over again because we haven't learnt what we needed to learn. Does this sound familiar?

Once a child has mastered walking, there are numerous other skills they have to learn. And that never ever stops. All that learning is enhanced by the information their mistakes give them. Kids just seem to know this, whereas most adults have forgotten.

Of course, when we finally learn what we need to learn, we just move on to the next mistake and growth opportunity. Which is why I have come to the conclusion that mistakes are the juice of life. Sometimes we have to repeat the same mistake over and over to finally learn the lesson.

Mistakes are often uncomfortable and can sometimes even be frightening. This can be because they reveal something about ourselves that we are not ready to see. Because that information scares us we tend to rationalise the mistake we've made as being someone or something else's fault, and therefore we miss the learning and growth opportunity. Blame always feels easier in the short-term.

But if we can summon the courage to look a little deeper into our mistake there is often vital information for us, and I have generally found that information to be freedom giving. Mistakes really are the keys to freedom. Think about that.

Activity – Mistakes

1. How do you feel once you've made a mistake?
2. What mistake have you just made that you could look at as a pathway to freedom, rather than as a tool to punish?

3. Can you think of a time when you made a mistake but then actually learnt something really valuable?

In order to learn the valuable lessons from our mistakes we have to let go of trying to be perfect and forgive ourselves.

1. In what ways do you try to be perfect?
2. How does that work out?
3. Do you feel happy once you have done something perfectly?
4. Could you do something right now that was just 'good enough', rather than perfect?

In order to let go of perfection I had to accept that there were some tasks that just needed to be done 'well enough'. I realised that by doing this I saved energy, I had less stress and when I looked at things objectively I saw that no one had noticed any difference, or even cared. It was also the start of being free from what other people thought of me. 'Good enough' and 'well enough' were good enough for me.

See where you can apply this in your own life. Pay attention to how you feel and try taking a step back to see what really matters. Does it matter that your family had a home cooked gourmet meal tonight or you just threw a few things together at the last minute? What is more important, the connection of just being with people you love or a perfectly set table and meal? If it's a special occasion maybe the home cooked meal is important, but if you are tired, sick or stressed it might be something you just can't achieve today.

When I get confused (and I still do) about where I really need to put in the effort, I ask myself this question: 'What will matter more in ten years?' This is a really effective and powerful question because the answer becomes clear very quickly. What matters more is that you are present and connected with the people you love – you will remember that in ten years, rather than what you ate. I use this question with my son all the time: 'What will matter more in ten years – that I finished doing the laundry or that I played trains with him because right now he really wants me to play trains?' So, horror of horrors, I leave the laundry half done and play trains with my son for half an hour. Because in ten years that bond we created will matter so much more than whether my laundry was folded.

What are you inviting into your experience?

Now we are going to move on to your goals in sobriety. By setting goals we are taking back control of the direction of our lives. Sobriety will give you the freedom to become the best version of yourself, rather than the worst.

For too long as alcoholics, we believe that we are victims of our circumstances. A common limiting belief is that if this bad stuff happened to you, you would drink too.

We think we can't change, we think we have no control over our lives, we believe it's all pointless and hopeless. That may be true when we are drinking but it's certainly not true when we are sober.

When we get sober we have the ability to choose what we invite into our experience. *We get to choose the experience we want.*

This was an outrageous concept to me when I first discovered it. How was it possible that I had invited in all the awful things that had happened to me? Over time I thought about it and realised that my thinking had been so negative and my self-esteem so low that my experience just matched my thinking.

But what about the abusive things that happen? When we have been abused or mistreated by other people through no fault of our own? When that is the case, we still have a choice in how we respond. We didn't choose the abuse, but we can choose our *response* to it.

In *Man's Search for Meaning*, Viktor Frankl discusses that no matter what we endure or suffer at the hands of others, we have absolute power in how we choose to respond to our suffering. This is very powerful stuff.

Victor Frankl discovered this when he was a Jewish prisoner in Auschwitz. The Nazis had taken from him everything it was possible to take, they had abused him and his family in unimaginable ways. On a daily basis he saw suffering that is beyond our comprehension. While he experienced this, he came to the conclusion that the one thing the Nazis could not touch were his mind and his thoughts. They were solely his and he could experience them however he chose.

He realised that even amongst the most unimaginable suffering it was possible to find meaning in life. He survived Auschwitz and went on to have a happy and successful life as an Existential Psychologist. He died in 1997.

When I'm struggling, or I get into a hole and everything seems bleak, I try to remember that I have a choice in how I respond to what is happening to me. It is immensely powerful to know this. Once I know this I can act on it and when I act from this perspective, my circumstances change. Everything starts flowing in the right direction again.

I learnt that life has its hurdles and sometimes they throw me off course and I feel powerless. But more and more I've learnt that I can choose what I invite into my experience, because I can choose my thoughts. My mind, and what I allow into it, is my responsibility.

Goals in sobriety

Now that you are sober it's time for you to take responsibility for the direction of your life. We are going to look at goals in all areas of your life. It's important to remember that we can make our own goals, and they should always be realistic. This is not an exercise to set ourselves up to fail so that we can then feel bad about ourselves. That is not productive. Goals are what we are aiming for. If we don't achieve them then we can look for feedback as to why that was. Not as a way to beat ourselves up, but as a way to learn and grow.

As human beings, we are made up of different components that all need to be fulfilled and explored. For example, we can have career goals but if our personal life is non-existent we are unlikely to be happy. The key here is balance.

We are going to be looking at goals in the following areas:
- Relationships: romantic relationships and friendships
- Social life
- Career/Education
- Physical health
- Emotional health
- Spiritual growth

Relationships

Let's look at relationships first. Now that you have done some work on relationships you will have a much better idea of what you want.

Activity – Romantic relationships

1. What is your goal in romantic relationships?
2. What do you need to do to get there?
3. What are your first steps?
4. What will success look like?

Activity – Friendships

1. What is your goal with your friendships?
2. What changes can you make right now?
3. What are the first steps you need to take for your friendship circle to look the way you want it to?
4. What does success look like?

Social life

If your social life was based around drinking then you are going to need to reinvent it. Because of our misconceptions about sobriety we can sometimes have this fear that our social life will be over and we will never have fun again. Nothing could be further from the truth. In time we will see that our previous social life was narrow and restricted. You may have things you've always wanted to do, but never got round to doing because you were always in a bar.

Activity – Social life

1. Make a list of things you've always wanted to do but drinking prevented you from doing.

2. Is there something on your list you could start doing now?
3. What would you like your social life to look like a year from now?

Career/Education

You may have a career right now, or you may not. You might have been just working for money so that you could afford to drink. Often the 'job' is the last thing to go for alcoholics. They will lose their relationships, driving licence, custody of their children before their job, because the job is where the money is and the money is where the alcohol is.

Activity – Career

1. A year from now how would you like to see your career? Does it include more education or finishing some education?
2. What are your passions career-wise?
3. What are the first steps in shaping your career/education goals?
4. What would success look like?

Physical health

If we drink to excess then we will have affected our health. When we become sober we have an opportunity for our bodies to heal from the excessive toxins we have been pouring into it. It's important to note that we shouldn't go overboard in this area (or any area). Whatever level your physical health is at right now it's important that you don't take things too far by embarking on an extreme diet or exercise plan – this is not something that would be good for your long-term sobriety.

Remember that the key to successful, sustainable sobriety is balance. If we focus too much on one goal then everything may get thrown out of balance. Sure, you could train really hard to get into the best physical shape possible and enter triathlons. But if all your time is spent exercising, what about your family and friendships, how will you nurture connections if you are always on a treadmill?

Activity – Physical health

1. What is your goal for your physical health?
2. Does this balance with your other goals?
3. What does success look like?

Emotional/Mental health

Equally as important as our physical health is our mental and emotional health. Think of it this way: if you brush your teeth, wash your face, take the stairs and eat your broccoli, then you are taking care of your physical health. What do you do to take care of your emotional well-being? Emotional well-being is very much about balance.

Activity – Mental health and emotional well-being

1. Are you getting enough sleep and rest?
2. Are you connecting with people and getting enough time alone?
3. Are you involved in activities that give you joy?
4. Do you have an outlet for your stresses and fears?
5. Who can you talk to who understands and doesn't judge you?
6. Is one of your goals this year to see a therapist or life coach and finally resolve those issues that have dogged you your whole life?
7. How do you define emotional well-being?
8. What do you need to do to support your mental health?
9. What are your next steps to bring balance into your life?
10. Describe how you would like to feel a year from now.

Spiritual growth

Very much tied to emotional and mental well-being is spiritual well-being.

People often get nervous when the subject of spirituality comes up. It can remind them of uncomfortable experiences they may have had with churches and religious leaders.

In *Why You Drink and How to Stop* I wrote:

Spirituality is not necessarily related to religion. It can be something else altogether, although confusingly it is the basis of *all* religions, if you accept that the explicit purpose of most religions is to take care of our 'souls'.

[To understand spirituality we must first understand what our 'spirit' actually is.]

Our spirit is the *real* us, the part not many other people see.

Our spirit is where our hopes, our dreams, our fears, our secrets, our shame, our joy exist.

[It is the conversation you have with yourself from the day you are born.]

It is our intuition, our gut instinct.

It is our sense of right and wrong.

Our spirit is intangible, *but we all know it's there.*

It's what makes you, you. And me, me.

Our spirit is unique to us. *It is us.*

How I feel about other people and the world around me comes from how my spirit responds.

When I love and appreciate my spirit is ignited. When I am hurt and broken my spirit is crushed.

When I die, for a while you can still touch my body, you can still see me. But I will be gone; my spirit – who I really was – will no longer be there.

You can't touch or hold or control my spirit.

It is me.

That is what our spirits are. Does that make sense? I'll give you an even simpler explanation of spirituality.

Spirituality is just being good to your spirit (your inner-self that no one else sees). *It is honouring who you really are.*

I want to be really clear about what spiritual health means: it's something that is very connected to your emotional well-being. It means taking care of your soul in a way that feels congruent for you. It may also mean trying something new and stepping out of your comfort zone.

Spirituality is all about connecting with *who you really are*. In active alcoholism we become 'fake' people; the way we behave when we are drinking is not representative of who we are. We need to reclaim our 'real' selves.

Activity – Spiritual growth

1. How do you define 'spiritual growth'?
2. What can you do to grow towards your definition?
3. What activities can you incorporate into your daily life that would be good for your spiritual growth? eg meditation, reading something empowering, quiet time

Restoring balance in our lives

I have mentioned 'balance' a lot and I cannot emphasise enough just how important it is to staying sober. Achieving balance in our life is something we need to be continuously paying attention to. Usually we will get some kind of 'red flag' that indicates we are ignoring a part of ourselves that needs care and attention. If I'm stressed and snippy at people it's a red flag that I'm not getting enough rest or that I'm working too hard. Maybe I have some uncomfortable feelings I haven't paid attention to and this is being manifested in my behaviour. Generally, if I am feeling out of sorts then I start by checking my balance. Am I doing too much of one thing and not enough of another?

The thing to learn about balance is that it changes over time. The circumstances of my life change and I have to adjust to how I balance my needs with these changes. Before I had children it was pretty easy to get exercise and to take care of my emotional and spiritual well-being. Being a mother of small children changed all that. So I had to adjust. I wasn't able to go to the gym every day and then go to a workshop on spirituality. So I had to re-think how I met my needs in these areas.

In many ways 'balance' is a moving target. As long as we are aware of it and become attuned to the signs that we need to adjust, life and sobriety become easier.

Activity – Balance

- What areas of my life are out of balance right now?
- What adjustment can I make?
- Are these realistic?
- What warning signs do I need to pay attention to?
- If my life were balanced in the next year what would it look like?

Maintaining your sobriety

If you have completed the exercises in this book then you will have learnt a lot about yourself and your drinking problem. The areas that have caused you problems should be clear to you now. From now on, you need to prioritise your sobriety and continue to 'work on yourself'. 'Working' on yourself is really just about doing things that empower you to grow into the best version of yourself, like keeping a check on your resentments and fears, listening to 'red flags' that indicate your balance is off and making conscious changes in your life.

Getting sober and staying sober are not isolated events. They require daily input. This can sound daunting but it really is nothing more than learning a new 'habit'. Consider how much of your time was taken up drinking, thinking about drinking and recovering from drinking. Did you spend twenty, forty, eighty hours per week on all that? Getting sober will certainly take up a lot of your time in the early days. Something that caused such destruction in your life can't be dealt with in just a few hours.

However, over time life becomes easier and all of these sober habits become a natural part of who you are. All of the things I do to maintain my sobriety and my spiritual/emotional wellbeing take a small amount of time. They don't feel like a chore as they are ingrained in me. Also, because I get very clear rewards from these practices I am incredibly incentivised to do them.

Let me put it this way: I am an alcoholic and it is in my nature to be all about the 'good stuff'. I drank because I thought 'good stuff' or 'good feelings' would then happen. If they did, of course they were only temporary. If these new behaviours didn't bring me 'good stuff', like feeling comfortable in my own skin, liking myself, feeling confident, dealing with people easily, then I would have given up long ago. There has to be a pay off.

I urge you to give this just a little bit of time and wait for the pay off ...

Activity – Staying sober

1. What do you need to do next?
2. What is your plan for the next thirty days to maintain your sobriety?
3. What is your plan for the next twelve months? What changes do you need to make?
4. Why do you want to stay sober?

Lastly ...

Thank you for reading this far. I am very proud of you for taking this massive step. I have been continuously sober since 2000. I have made a lot of mistakes along the way but I've never needed to drink to cope with any of them. There have been challenges and joys but I wouldn't change a thing. I am who I am today because of my recovery from alcoholism.

These are some of the most important things I have learnt so far:
1. Just when you think you've nailed it ...
   More than once I've thought 'I've got this!', 'I know everything there is to know about recovery and addiction', 'I've dealt with all my issues – I don't really need to do any more work on myself'. Yes, that usually happens right before I fall flat on my ass.
2. The growth never stops.
   It smooths out a lot. Things are definitely less bumpy. But there is always more to know and if you think you know all there is to know, then see above.
3. We teach other people how to treat us.
   My behaviour will instruct you on whether to walk all over me, abuse me or hurt me. Instead, I can teach you how to treat me, with the boundaries I protect and by saying what I mean.

4. Say what you mean, mean what you say.
   People do not need to hear me waffling on about my story; they do not need excuses. They generally just need a truthful 'yes' or 'no'. My life became so much simpler and calmer when I learnt how to do this.

5. I have to take responsibility for the experience I want to have.
   By practising the above I become responsible for the experience I am having right now. If events or circumstances are out of my control then I always get to choose my response. Therefore I am responsible for my experience, in all circumstances, without fail.

6. If you don't do the work, the shine will go off your recovery.
   Being sober is just not enough. I need more than that. If I don't put the work in, then I may stay sober, but I'll stop feeling comfortable in my own skin. I'll drift back to being discontented and fearful.

7. Give it away to keep it.
   When my life came together in sobriety and my career and personal life went well I forgot to work with newcomers. Don't do that. Giving of yourself is actually what fills your tanks.

8. Does this (whatever it is) always need to be said, and does it need to be said by you?
   Not usually, I have discovered. Only give your opinion if explicitly asked. Believe me, it saves a lot of time and trouble.

9. Exercise.
   Of all the things I have just told you, this is the most important one. The benefits of exercise on your emotional well-being outweigh everything else you can possibly do.

10. Practise listening.
    None of us listens well. Quiet the noise in your head and really focus on what people are saying. You will be amazed at what you hear.

11. It was never about you.
    What a relief! It was never about me anyway. What *you* did or said had nothing at all to do with my life. Everyone else is wrapped up in their own stuff too. Now I can stop worrying what other people think and get on with it!

12. Nothing is ever personal.

    See above. What other people do, say or think is always about them, not me. Even when it seems like it is, what other people do or say always, without fail, comes through the filters of their own experience, values and judgement. Therefore it is not personal to me but a simple expression of how they feel at that particular time. It took me a while to get that one.

13. The journey is joyous.

    Life is not about the destination but the journey. We are always in a state of becoming the best version of ourselves. Uncovering who we really are is the point of it all. All I ever had to do was just keep moving.

14. Love well.

    There was always much love here for me – I just refused to see it for a while. Always choose love. The choices I have made in my life based on fear have never worked out. If I choose love, then things don't always work out the way I want or planned but man, is the adventure a good one!

Printed in Great Britain
by Amazon